Revolutionary Doctors

Revolutionary Doctors

*How Venezuela and Cuba Are Changing the World's
Conception of Health Care*

by STEVE BROUWER

MONTHLY REVIEW PRESS
New York

Library of Congress Cataloging-in-Publication Data

Brouwer, Steve, 1947–

Revolutionary doctors : how Venezuela and Cuba are changing the world's conception of health care / by Steve Brouwer.

p. ; cm.

Includes bibliographical references and index.

ISBN 978-1-58367-239-6 (pbk. : alk. paper) — ISBN 978-1-58367-240-2 (cloth : alk. paper) 1. Community health services—Venezuela. 2. Community health services—Cuba. 3. Medical education—Venezuela. 4. Medical education—Cuba. I. Title.

[DNLM: 1. Community Health Services—Cuba. 2. Community Health Services—Venezuela. 3. Education, Medical—methods—Cuba. 4. Education, Medical—methods—Venezuela. 5. Health Services Accessibility—Cuba. 6. Health Services Accessibility—Venezuela. 7. International Cooperation—Cuba. 8. International Cooperation—Venezuela. 9. Physicians—Cuba. 10. Physicians—Venezuela. 11. Poverty—Cuba. 12. Poverty—Venezuela. WA 546 DV4]

RA481.B76 2011

362.109-7291—dc23

2011016108

Monthly Review Press

146 West 29th Street, Suite 6W

New York, NY 10001

5 4 3 2 1

Contents

Acknowledgments

I did not go to Venezuela in September of 2007 to write a book about the revolutionary practice of medicine. I went to live in a mountain village and write about how rural people, especially the campesinos in and around Monte Carmelo, were transforming their lives through their active participation in the Bolivarian Revolution. Although I narrowed my focus to tell about one important part of this revolutionary process and its connection to the Cuban Revolution, I learned an immense amount about rural life from my campesino neighbors in Monte Carmelo, who provided support, kindness, and friendship to me and my sons during our nine-month stay. This small village is gaining renown throughout Venezuela for its cooperative spirit, solidarity, experimental agriculture, and grassroots organizing ability, and so it really merits a book of its own. (I hope to write more about Monte Carmelo. In the meantime, readers can still find blog articles I wrote in 2007–08 at www.venezuelanotes.blogspot.com.)

Though I cannot possibly list the names of everyone who ought to be thanked, I want to give special thanks to the family of Gaudy and Omar Garcia and the family of Abigail and Gabriel Garcia, and other members of their extended families: Sandino, Luz Marina, Polilla, Carmen Alicia, Hector, Alexis, Arturo, Cesar, Javier, and Maira. They not only provided us with hospitality, close friendship, and a place to live but were invaluable in sharing an intimate knowledge of village life, farming, and the beautiful natural world that surrounds them.

I am especially indebted to the medical students and doctors in the Monte Carmelo and Sanare area who allowed me to spend time in their clinics and classrooms, as well as learn about their lives and aspirations. I refer to them only by their first names since I do not have everyone's last name accurately recorded. The Venezuelan medical students: Mariela, Milena, Édison, Jonás, Arelys, Iris, Yeiny, Inez, Odalys, Luisa, Antonio, Magaly, Vanesa, Dilbex, José, Hilario, Rosana, Mileidy, Vanesa, Karina, Juan, and José Antonio; the students from Suriname: Georgo, Isabel, and Meredith. Doctors working at the Barrio Adentro walk-in clinics and the Diagnostic Center: Dr. Tomasa, Dr. Barbara, Dr. Edita, Dr. Raúl, the two Dr. Franks, Dr. Alina, and Dr. Humberto.

Many thanks to two North American friends, Lisa Sullivan and Charlie Hardy, who have lived for decades in Venezuela, spending most of that time living and working among the poor in the barrios of Caracas and Barquisimeto. They were indispensable for introductions to many Venezuelans who became friends and contacts, and invaluable in their help on various trips I made to Venezuela.   Five friends from the nearby town of Sanare, all of them teachers—Honorio, Irlanda, Rubén, Goya, and Luis—were particularly helpful in acquainting me with local progressive and revolutionary traditions in education, politics, religion, and society that predate the Chávez government institutions. The two Morochos, the unofficial village anthropologists and poets of Monte Carmelo, were very generous in filling me in on local history and folklore. My first guides to Caracas, Marcela and Antonio, gave me an exceptional introduction to the barrios and the rest of the city. Other valued friends who helped in Venezuela include Mario, Rosa Elena, Pablo, Ledys, David, Pachi, Maia, Joséito, and Father Mario Grippo.

In Cuba, my good friends the poet Victor Casaus and journalist Hedelberto Lopez Blanch were extremely helpful in Havana. Gail Reed and Conner Gorry, journalists based in Havana working for

MEDICC Review, provided me with invaluable advice and information. *MEDICC Review*, featuring articles by Cuban and U.S. medical experts, is the only peer-reviewed journal in English dedicated to Cuban medicine. This magazine and website, a joint venture by Cuban and U.S. medical experts, is a great resource and extremely reliable. I want to thank philosopher and journalist Enrique Ubieta Gómez for sharing his time with me and thoughts related to his excellent book, *Venezuela rebelde: dinero vs. solidaridad*. At ELAM, the Latin American School of Medicine in Havana, Dr. Midalys Castilla Martínez, the vice rector, was generous with her time as she introduced me to the school and some of the students.

At Monthly Review Press, I would like to thank Fred Magdoff, who visited us briefly in Venezuela and suggested the press could be interested in a book on revolutionary medicine. Michael Yates has been an excellent editor, displaying great patience and sound judgment, and Erin Clermont served as a great copyeditor with a sharp eye for clarity.

My two sons, Jan and Ari, who were eighteen and sixteen at the time, lived with me in Monte Carmelo and provided wonderful companionship and good humor. They also ended up working full-time with our campesino neighbors at the Las Lajitas cooperative organic farm—they began their half-hour climb up the mountain at 5:30 every morning and spent their days digging, planting, harvesting, and composting with worms; they even learned how to plow with a horse on the steep mountainsides. In the afternoons they came home with an extraordinary variety of vegetables and the world's tastiest yogurt. And many thanks, as always, to my wife, Susan, who could only visit us for a few weeks because she had to stay at home in Pennsylvania teaching her classes while providing lots of encouragement, love, and our material support.

Finally I want to dedicate this book to the memory of my father, Dr. Stephen W. Brouwer, a physician renowned for his good humor and willingness to listen to patients. One of the few things that could anger him was the death of someone who sought treatment too late because of worries about the cost. He blamed such deaths on a health system that would not countenance free and universal care. My father was the only doctor I knew in my youth who was a socialist—in fact, he was the only socialist I knew—so he would surely be glad to know that today revolutionary doctors are transforming health care in the poorest and most remote parts of the Americas.

1. Where Do Revolutionary Doctors Come From?

The campesinos would have run, immediately and with unreserved enthusiasm, to help their brothers.
—CHE GUEVARA, "On Revolutionary Medicine," 1960

Even though he came to Cuba with a rifle slung over his shoulder and entered Havana in 1959 as one of the victorious commanders of the Cuban Revolution, he still continued to think of himself as a doctor. Five years earlier, the twenty-five-year-old Argentine had arrived in Guatemala and offered to put his newly earned medical degree at the service of a peaceful social transformation. Dr. Ernesto Guevara was hoping to find work in the public health services and contribute to the wide-ranging reforms being initiated by President Arbenz, but he never had much opportunity to work as a physician in Guatemala. Within months of his arrival, Arbenz's government was brought down by the military coup d'état devised by the United Fruit Company, some Guatemalan colonels, the U.S. State Department, and the CIA.

Che never lost sight of the value of his original aspiration—combining the humanitarian mission of medicine with the creation of a just society. When he addressed the Cuban militia on August 19, 1960, a year and a half after the triumph of the revolution, he chose to speak about "Revolutionary Medicine" and the possibility of educating a new kind of doctor.

> A few months ago, here in Havana, it happened that a group of newly graduated doctors did not want to go into the country's rural areas and demanded remuneration before they would agree to go. . . .
>
> But what would have happened if instead of these boys, whose families generally were able to pay for their years of study, others of less fortunate means had just finished their schooling and were beginning the exercise of their profession? What would have occurred if two or three hundred campesinos had emerged, let us say by magic, from the university halls?
>
> What would have happened, simply, is that the campesinos would have run, immediately and with unreserved enthusiasm, to help their brothers.

Since then, Cuban medicine and health services have been developed in a number of unique and revolutionary ways, but only now, nearly fifty years later, has Che's dream come to full fruition. Today it is literally true that campesinos, along with the children of impoverished working-class and indigenous communities, are becoming doctors and running, "with unreserved enthusiasm, to help their brothers."

While this is happening on the mountainsides of Haiti, among the Garifuna people on the Caribbean coast of Honduras, in the villages of Africa and the highlands of Bolivia, it is occurring on the grandest scale in the rural towns and city barrios of Venezuela. When I was living in the mountains of western Venezuela in 2007 and 2008, I witnessed the emergence of revolutionary doctors every morning as I walked out the door of our little tin-roofed house. The scene would have delighted Che:

> As the sun rises above the mountain behind the village of Monte Carmelo and the white mist begins to lift off the cloud forest, four young campesinos walk along the road in their wine-red polo shirts

with their crisp, white jackets folded up under their arms to protect them from the dust. At 7 a.m. they wave goodbye to the high school students who are waiting to begin their classes in three rooms at the women's cooperative and then hop aboard the "taxi," a tough, thirty-year-old Toyota pickup truck that often packs twenty or more people in the back. They travel down the winding mountain road, through the deep ravine at the bottom, and up the hill on the far side of the valley to the larger town of Sanare, where they are going to work all morning alongside Cuban doctors in neighborhood consulting offices and the modern Diagnostic Clinic.

Around 7:45, four more medical students from the village, already donning their white jackets, walk by our house, past the plaza and the little church, and gather in front of a small concrete block building called the *ambulatorio*. About the same time, they are joined by three more medical students who emerge from Carlos's bright blue jeep, "the Navigator," one of the other vehicles in the taxi cooperative that serves the village. These students from Sanare pull on their white jackets, hug their compañeros, and wait for Elsy, a health committee volunteer who is studying to be a nurse, to unlock the gate to the *ambulatorio*, the walk-in clinic that offers Barrio Adentro medical service.

As I stroll by, I see the prospective patients sitting on the benches of the small, covered patio in front of the entrance door. They are waiting for Dr. Tomasa, the family medical specialist. Two chirpy teenage girls sit next to Dr. Raul's dentistry room and grin with perfect-looking smiles. "What could be wrong with your teeth?" I ask.

"Nothing," responds one of them, "Dr. Raul is giving us another checkup." Another checkup? Their parents never had a single checkup when they were young—consequently, there are many people over forty or fifty who have very few teeth.

By 8 a.m. one of the medical students stands behind the simple wooden counter, performing receptionist duties. Another shuttles back and forth to the file shelves, organizing and updating medical information that is kept on every family in the community. A third chats informally with the waiting patients, entertaining their small children, and informally inquiring about their families' health. The other four students stand alongside Dr. Tomasa in the consulting office, watching her take family and individual histories and give examinations. They also fetch medicines, take temperatures, and weigh healthy children who are accompanying their mothers. Today, like every day, Dr. Tomasa says to her students, "*Por favor,* more questions. This is how we learn. You can never ask too many questions."

Monte Carmelo is a small village that stretches along a single paved road on a mountain ridge in the foothills of the Andes in the state of Lara. Before Hugo Chávez assumed the presidency of Venezuela in 1999, the road was unpaved and the high school did not exist. According to the 2007 census, its population consisted of 129 families and approximately 700 individuals, nearly all of them supporting themselves by working small parcels of land by hand, or with horses and oxen. That same year nine residents of Monte Carmelo were medical students. Eight were studying Medicina Integral Comunitaria (popularly known as MIC), an intensive six-year course that in English is usually called Comprehensive Community Medicine. A ninth village resident was studying medicine in Cuba. Two more young women from a neighboring hamlet were also in medical school. They were part of a group of sixty-seven students in this agricultural region who were becoming doctors of medicine.

The students are a diverse lot: some are nineteen or twenty years old and have recently finished high school; others are closer to thirty and have young children; a few are even older. Some young mothers have recently completed their secondary education through Mission Ribas, one of the Bolivarian social missions that bring adults back to school on evenings and weekends. All of the students are enthusiastic about their role in fostering good health and introducing reliable medical care into the fabric of their community and the larger world. And many of them dream of emulating their Cuban teachers and one day serving as internationalist physicians themselves in remote and impoverished parts of the world.

This experiment in training new doctors in MIC would be worthy of international attention even if the program was limited to the 67 students in this remote coffee-growing region in the state of Lara. But in fact they represent only a tiny fraction of a gigantic effort to transform medical education and health care delivery throughout all of Venezuela. Nearly 25,000 students were enrolled in the first four years of MIC in 2007–2008, and by 2009 and 2010 they were joined by more students, swelling the ranks of students enrolled in all six years of MIC to approximately 30,000. This is almost as many as the total number of doctors who were practicing medicine in all capacities in Venezuela when Hugo Chávez was elected president in 1998.

One unique aspect of MIC is that the students in Monte Carmelo do not have to leave the *campo,* the countryside, nor do students in the poorest neighborhoods of Venezuelan cities have to desert their barrios in order to attend medical school. Medicina Integral Comunitaria is a "university without walls" that trains young doctors in their home environments. This is not a short-term course for health aides or "barefoot doctors," but a rigorous program designed to produce a new kind of physician. Every morning during their years of study, the MIC students help doctors working in Barrio Adentro attend to patients' illnesses and learn to comprehend the broad public health needs of their communities. And every afternoon, they meet with their MIC professors in a series of formal medical classes that constitute a rigorous curriculum and include all the medical sciences studied at traditional universities.

The MIC education program could not exist without Barrio Adentro, the nationwide health system that first began delivering primary care in 2003 thanks to an enormous commitment of expertise from Cuba. From 2004 to 2010, Barrio Adentro continually deployed between 10,000 and 14,000 Cuban doctors and 15,000 to 20,000 other Cuban medical personnel—dentists, nurses, physical therapists, optometrists, and technicians. Their services are available to all Venezuelans for free at almost 7,000 walk-in offices and over 500 larger diagnostic clinics, and they have been very effective in meeting the needs of 80 percent of the population that had been ill-served or not served at all by the old health care system.

Obviously, Cuba cannot afford to devote so many of its medical personnel to Venezuela indefinitely, nor does the Chávez government want to depend on foreign doctors forever. So when Barrio Adentro was being launched in 2003, Cuban and Venezuelan medical experts devised a new program of medical education that will enable Venezuela to keep its universal public health program functioning permanently. Starting in 2005, the Cuban doctors were asked to perform a rigorous double duty: not only did they continue treating patients in Barrio Adentro clinics, but many of them also began teaching as professor/tutors for the MIC program in comprehensive community medicine. The goal of MIC is to integrate the training of family practitioners into the fabric of communities in a holistic effort that meets the medical needs of all citizens, makes use of local resources, and promotes preventive health care and healthy living.

The Cuban mission in Venezuela is possible because over the past half-century, Cuba has developed a vision of medical service that goes far beyond its own borders. Cuban health workers, in addition to providing free health care for all their fellow citizens, have transformed themselves into a "weapon of solidarity," a revolutionary force that has been deployed in over 100 countries around the world. Since 2000, however, the Cuban commitment has increased substantially because the Bolivarian Revolution in Venezuela has contributed its own enthusiasm, volunteers, and economic resources. Through various agreements of cooperation, Cuba and Venezuela have embarked upon a number of projects in other fields such as education, agriculture, energy, and industrial development, and then have extended these cooperative ventures to other nations, particularly within ALBA, the Bolivarian Alliance for the Peoples of Our America, which includes Bolivia, Nicaragua, and Ecuador as well as the small Caribbean island nations of Dominica, Antigua and Barbuda, Saint Vincent and the Grenadines.

Of all these ambitious undertakings, delivering medical services is by far the most prominent. In order to extend universal health care to the poor and working classes in way that is compatible with the new, egalitarian vision of these societies, many more physicians are needed. With this in mind, Cuba is educating more doctors at home even as it trains tens of thousands in Venezuela. In 2008 there were 29,000 Cubans enrolled in medical school, plus nearly 24,000 foreign students (including more than one hundred students from the United States) studying at the Latin American School of Medicine in Havana or at the schools of the New Program for the Training of Latin American Doctors that are located in four other provinces.

An Army in White Jackets

I first became aware of the magnitude of this medical revolution in 2004 on my first trip to Venezuela. When Dr. Yonel, a young Cuban dentist working in a barrio of Caracas, informed me there were more than 10,000 doctors working in Venezuela, I exclaimed, "*Un ejército de medicos!* An army of doctors!"

Dr. Yonel smiled and replied, "*Un ejército de paz. A*n army of peace."

Clearly the collaboration of the rejuvenated Cuban Revolution and the nascent Bolivarian Revolution was yielding impressive results. And a growing number of countries in the Western Hemisphere, long under the yoke of wealthy conservative minorities or military authoritarians who were dependent on capital and political instruction from the North, were no longer willing to listen to the United States when it told them to shun Cuba and Venezuela. Since its long-standing economic blockade of Cuba was failing to deter these developments, the United States tried to launch a disruptive dissident movement in Cuba and assist a coup d'état in Venezuela. When these efforts failed, the U.S. government imposed more draconian economic and travel restrictions on Cuba in 2004 and funded various schemes to undermine both revolutionary governments. In 2006, the United States stooped to an especially low level when it attempted to directly sabotage Cuba's humanitarian medical missions by creating the Cuban Medical Professional Parole Program. This was a law specifically designed to lure Cuban doctors, nurses, and technicians away from their foreign assignments by offering them special immigration status and speedy entry into the United States.

These antagonistic efforts did not succeed in diminishing the international solidarity and prestige that Cuba and Venezuela were acquiring around the world, nor did it keep them from expanding their programs of humanitarian medical aid and international medical education. In 2007, a young Chilean, a member of the third class graduating from the Latin American School of Medicine in Havana, spoke at her commencement and told her classmates: "Today we are an army in white jackets that will bring good health and a little more dignity to our people."[1]

By 2010, Cuba and Venezuela further demonstrated their capabilities by being among the most prominent providers of both emergency and long-term aid to Haiti after its devastating earthquake. Brazil, the economic giant of Latin America, signaled its admiration by announcing that it would be delighted to join Cuba in a partnership to create a new public health system in Haiti. José Gomés, the Brazilian Minister of Health, explained why his country was choosing to work with the Cubans on such a significant and demanding project: "We have just signed an agreement—Cuba, Brazil, and Haiti—according to which all three countries make a commitment to unite our forces in order to reconstruct the health system in Haiti. . . . We will provide this, together with Cuba—a country with an extremely long internationalist experience, a great degree of technical ability, great determination, and an enormous amount of heart."[2]

For Cuba, Venezuela, and by extension their allies in ALBA alliance, these triumphs throughout the first decade of the twenty-first century were more than diplomatic coups, they were moral victories. They demonstrated the power of social solidarity and humanistic concern for other people, values in stark contrast with the materialistic, self-centered, and aggressive behavior of the advanced capitalist societies.

This book aims to acquaint the reader with the ways that revolutionary doctors and health care workers have developed into major protagonists of socialist change and are defining what that change should look like. Chapters 2 through 4 offer some glimpses of Cu. international medical missions, their profound impact on variou parts of the world, and their relation to the overall development of Cuban health care over the past fifty years. Chapters 5 through 8 describe how a new public health system, Barrio Adentro, has been created in Venezuela, and how new Venezuelan doctors are being educated to assume responsibility for this system in the future. This description is based on my own observations of day-to-day interactions of doctors, medical students, health committees, and the members of the communities they serve. Finally, the last four chapters illustrate how capitalist cultures and imperialist forces are resisting the development of revolutionary medicine and revolutionary consciousness, while the emerging socialist cultures are pressing forward with new ideas and creating the patterns of practice and commitment in daily life that are producing the revolutionaries of the future.

2. Solidarity and Internationalism

> I began to travel throughout America . . . First as a student and later as a doctor, I came into close contact with poverty, hunger, and disease; with the inability to treat a child because of lack of money; with the stupefaction provoked by continual hunger and punishment, to the point that a father can accept the loss of a son as an unimportant accident, as occurs often in the downtrodden classes of our American homeland. And I began to realize at that time that there were things that were almost as important to me as becoming famous or making a significant contribution to medical science: I wanted to help those people.
>
> —CHE GUEVARA, "On Revolutionary Medicine," 1960 speech

Che's travels through the American hemisphere in the early 1950s were his first steps toward developing a revolutionary international consciousness. Over the next few years his desire to help the poor and the oppressed was transformed into a decision to stand in solidarity with them, and to join in their struggles to assert their dignity and humanity. When he arrived in Guatemala hoping to put his medical skills at the service of the people, there were no Latin American networks that promoted internationalism and solidarity on the part of young health professionals who wanted to work and live among the poorest people in the hemisphere.

Today there is such a place, founded in 1998, which bears this inscription on the walls of its reception hall:

ESTA SERÁ UNA BATALLA DE LA SOLIDARIDAD CONTRA EL EGOÍSMO.
(This will be a battle of solidarity against selfishness.)

The quotation from Fidel can be found inside the Latin American School of Medicine outside Havana (in Spanish the school is called La Escuela Latinoamericana de Medicina, usually referred to by its acronym, ELAM). Fidel's words are written in oversized script above a large map of the world that indicates all the places where Cuban medical brigades have completed humanitarian missions through a program of international medical cooperation known as Plan Integral de Salud (the Comprehensive Health Plan). The school, like the inscription, is a testimony to Che's vision and to the example set by the Cuban health care professionals. By embracing the solidarity of international cooperation and offering free medical attention to everyone, they represent the ideal of service for the foreign students who come to ELAM.

On other large maps in the entry hall at the medical school, there are lists of the exact number of students in attendance from twenty different countries. The large majority are the first in their families to attend any kind of university and come from poor communities that do not have adequate medical facilities. The students' obligation, in return for the free education they are receiving, is to return home in solidarity with the poor of their native country and dedicate themselves to practicing community health care and preventive medicine.

In March 2009, when I visited ELAM in Havana (there is also another much smaller ELAM campus in Santiago de Cuba, with students from five countries, including Haiti), there were 1,576 first-year students at the campus and another 1,287 in the second year of the six-year program. The rest of the 5,310 ELAM students, in their third through sixth years of studies, were continuing their training at other medical faculties located in all thirteen provinces of Cuba. The largest number of first-year students, 144, came from Mexico; next were 108 from Bolivia; way down the list, second to last in number, 27 from Belize; and finally, 23 students from the United States.

U.S. Students at the Latin American School of Medicine

Four of the U.S. students chatted with me when they had some free time between classes. One, Pasha Jackson, had an unusual personal history for an ELAM student, for he did not, like most students, come directly to Cuba from a poor family in an impoverished part of the hemisphere. He had come from the world of professional football. Pasha had played at the University of Oklahoma, then in the National Football League with the San Francisco 49ers, the Indianapolis Colts, and the Oakland Raiders. Nagged by a recurring shoulder injury during his four-year pro career, he finally decided to retire from the game. "It wasn't so difficult," he said, "because I had dreamt about two things all my life, being a football player and being a doctor. Now I could proceed with becoming a doctor."

Why did he come to Cuba? "I was looking for a revolutionary path in medicine, a way of becoming a physician and a revolutionary who can serve the people in the most helpful way possible. Medical school in the States didn't offer me that possibility. They are producing a different kind of M.D. It was my father who heard about studying medicine in Cuba and urged me to apply."

Frances, whose family comes from Nigeria, grew up in the South Bronx in New York City. She had finished her undergraduate studies and a year of postgraduate predoctoral courses in preparation for medical school, when she heard about the possibility of studying in Cuba from the pastor at her church. She said she had previously thought of applying to U.S. schools—"the University of Pennsylvania had an integrated curriculum that I particularly liked"—but they were prohibitively expensive. In 2009, she and Pasha were completing their premed year, an important preparatory course of study that gets all students on the same page and includes intensive language courses for non-Spanish-speaking students. In order to immerse herself more fully in the language, Francis had chosen to move out of her original dormitory area, which housed English-speaking students from the United States and Belize, and reside with all-Spanish-speaking students.

Ian Fabian, a Dominican American who also came from New York City, was in his first year of regular medical studies at ELAM in 2009. When he finished his undergraduate work and was working at a university neuroscience laboratory in New York, he too began thinking about applying to medical schools. The cost seemed very high to him, especially when he took note of the kinds of medical students who came through his laboratory. "Those students are super-competitive and individualistic. It's a cutthroat atmosphere, with no signs of a cooperative spirit and working together. I wanted something very different, an atmosphere of contributing together, helping each other along, working toward a common goal of serving society. When I heard about the possibility of studying here, I knew it was for me."

Malik Sharif, another first-year student, was also working at a laboratory, in his hometown of Cleveland, but like the others was discouraged about the cost of attending medical school and the overwhelming burden of taking out loans that could easily add up to $150,000 or $200,000. One day a medical school professor from Berkeley visited his lab, spoke highly of the quality of education available at ELAM, and suggested that Malik consider studying in Cuba. By working through the Interfaith Interreligious Foundation for Community Organizing founded by Reverend Lucius Walker of New York, Malik found that he could file an online application to ELAM in a very efficient and straightforward manner. Once in Cuba, Malik said, he and his fellow Americans were pleased to find it was not difficult to make adjustments to living in a different society. "And you know, it may seem like a small thing, but I was afraid I wouldn't like the food. The cafeteria people have looked after us very well." He was referring not only to the quality of the food, but to the fact that he and Pasha try to follow a Muslim diet. The cafeterias at ELAM cater to those who have special food needs, either for health or religious reasons. This way the two young men could avoid eating pork, one of the favorite meats of Cubans.

These four students were looking forward to practicing family medicine within a community setting, and wanted to find a way to integrate that practice into a social network of preventive care and promoting good health when they return to the United States. They know that family and community practice is not as well compensated as other specialties in U.S. medicine, but they said the lower pay ought to be sufficient for their needs, especially since they will not have huge loans to pay off like so many of their American counterparts.

Dr. Midalys Castilla Martínez, the vice rector in charge of instruction at ELAM, explained that there is no ideological test for incoming students, who are of various political persuasions and religious backgrounds; the latter are helped to find places where they can practice their religion while they are in Cuba.

Over time ELAM has devised ways to make this wide array of foreign students comfortable during their time in Cuba, and consequently the student retention rate in 2009 was 85 percent or more, about 10 percent higher than it used to be. The first year is the most difficult, and once students have managed to get into second year and beyond the retention rate is above 90 percent. The school realizes that all students are going to be separated from their own cultures for a very long time, so it provides various kinds of support. Dr. Castilla said that counselors and psychologists are available to talk with students about personal and social problems that arise. Furthermore, students are assigned *guias* or guides, faculty mentor/advisors who talk with them often and are aware of their academic progress and their personal demeanor, so that they will notice if a student is depressed, frustrated, or falling behind. Special tutoring is always available, so that any who are anxious about their progress or comprehension can get immediate help.

When it comes to the student's commitment to returning home to work with the neglected and excluded communities, Dr. Castilla acknowledged that there was no way for Cuba to enforce such a provision. However, ELAM has tried to work with progressive groups and government ministries in other countries to facilitate internships and entrée into public service. For a number of countries, such as Guatemala and Haiti, Cuba and ELAM have made agreements to establish formal residencies in comprehensive community medicine for graduates. Young Guatemalan and Haitian doctors return home and go to work in clinics in the remote rural areas where Cuban doctors have been working for more than a decade, preparing to assume this responsibility in the future. These residency programs, like ELAM itself, are a direct outgrowth of the Comprehensive Health Plan of 1998. In the United States, there is no public support for students returning from ELAM; in fact, the Bush administration would have barred all students from attending medical school in Cuba in 2004 if not for the intervention of Secretary of State Colin Powell, who argued that the U.S. government would face criticism for keeping a number of minority students from receiving a free medical education.

The Birth of Plan Integral de Salud

The campus of ELAM was once the Cuban Naval Academy, a place where both navy military recruits and merchant marine sailors were trained in the past. Its solid white buildings, trimmed in blue, sit in a picturesque location on the edge of the sea on the north coast of Cuba west of Havana. In 1998, according to Dr. Castilla, General Raúl Castro, then in charge of the Cuban armed forces, was overseeing the decommissioning of various military facilities throughout Cuba because the nation was committed to substantially reducing its military budget. He suggested to his brother, President Fidel Castro, that the Cuban naval academy would be an ideal location for a new medical school that would serve foreign students from Latin America. The conversion was approved in November of 1998, and the first students were able to enroll and attend classes in the latter part of 1999.

The sudden transformation of the Naval Academy into a medical school followed immediately upon the creation of the Plan Integral de

Salud, or Comprehensive Health Plan, that was Cuba's response to two devastating hurricanes, George and Mitch, that swept through the Caribbean and Central America in 1998. George struck Haiti and the Dominican Republic in the summer, and Mitch caused devastating floods and killed 30,000 people in Nicaragua, Belize, Guatemala, and Honduras in October 1998. Many of the areas most damaged by these disasters were remote places where people had little or no access to health services of any kind. Cuba immediately sent 2,000 doctors and other medical personnel to give emergency care for victims of the disasters, but they also offered another kind of commitment that proved even more valuable.

The Plan Integral de Salud is an agreement that promises free Cuban medical assistance over the long term to help rectify the deficiencies of local health systems. There are three main conditions in the agreement between Cuba and the host country:

1. The host country accepts Cuban medical collaborators, including doctors in comprehensive general medicine (*medicina general integral*), nurses, and other professionals, who stay for two-year periods and then are replaced by a new volunteers;

2. Cuban health care personnel not only provide primary health care to the local population but also start developing local human resources that will be able to promote good health care in the future. This includes onsite training of health assistants and grassroots educators in preventive medicine, as well as enrollment of young people at ELAM for a six-year medical education as physicians;

3. Cuban medical teams avoid interfering with the medical practices of local doctors; usually the teams are located in rural areas where no one has ever provided health care.

Cuba has been faithful to these accords, which rapidly spread beyond the Central American and Caribbean victims of the 1998 hurricanes, so that ten years later the Plan Integral de Salud included service to thirty-six different countries in Africa, Asia, Oceana, Latin America, and the Caribbean. At the end of 2008, there were 3,462 collaborators, 2,393 of them doctors, working on these missions. Because new medical personnel are rotated into these nations on a regular basis, the cumulative total of Cubans involved is very high. Approximately 67,000 health professionals worked in the Plan Integral de Salud missions between 1998 and 2008, over 6,000 of them in Haiti alone.

Because Cuba never planned on staying in the host nations forever, the Latin American School of Medicine was conceived and put into operation as soon as the first medical brigades were dispatched in 1998. In the first several years of ELAM's existence, the largest numbers of students enrolling and graduating with medical degrees came from three of the countries—Haiti, Guatemala, and Honduras—that originally agreed to take part in the Plan Integral de Salud. Now that ELAM has produced about 9,000 physicians who graduated in the first six classes (2005 through 2010), each of these countries has several hundred new doctors prepared to provide care to their underserved populations.

Cuban Support for Haiti

The significance of the Cuban commitment to international solidarity in health care can be appreciated by looking at the medical situation in Haiti on January 12, 2010. At the moment the monstrous earthquake shattered this nation, there were fewer than 2,000 Haitian doctors for a population of nine million people. In many parts of the country the only medical care available before the earthquake was being delivered by 344 Cuban medical professionals who were deployed on medical missions through the Plan Integral de Salud (more than half were physicians, the others highly trained nurses and medical technicians). They were working in public hospitals and small public clinics alongside Haitian medical personnel, many of whom had graduated from ELAM (547 Haitians obtained medical degrees from ELAM between 2005 and 2009).[1]

The core group of Cuban-trained medical workers quickly mobilized on the day after the earthquake, relocating as necessary to the hardest-hit areas, including the capital of Port-au-Prince. With 400 of the Haitian graduates from ELAM working with them, they proved to be the largest, most reliable, and best organized source of emergency treatment in the nation. Within a few weeks, 185 Haitian medical students from Cuba were also able to join the group as interns, granted leaves of absence from their fifth and sixth years of study at ELAM to aid their suffering nation.

This added up to a coordinated medical presence of nearly a thousand Cubans and Haitians who were familiar with Haiti's culture and Creole, the language of the vast majority of local citizens. Speaking both Creole and Spanish, this group was well equipped to translate for the rapidly growing contingents of Cuban-educated and Spanish-speaking doctors who kept arriving in Haiti. Over the course of the spring and the summer, the number of doctors who had been trained in Cuba kept expanding, so that by July they numbered over 1,500 and included ELAM graduates from Haiti and twenty-six other countries.

Also among those who recently graduated from ELAM were those who came in February to join the Henry Reeve Brigade. This was the first time that ELAM graduates had been incorporated into this prestigious group, which is composed of veteran Cuban medical experts who regularly respond to natural disasters throughout the world. The Henry Reeve Medical Brigade was named in honor of a nineteen-year-old American who volunteered to fight for Cuban independence in the Ten Years War of 1868–1878. Henry Reeve led cavalry troops against the Spanish army in over 400 engagements and injured his leg so badly that he had to be fitted with metal braces and strapped to his horse in order to ride into battle. He ended up a brigadier general under the command of the revolutionary hero General Máximo Gómez, and died when his cavalry unit was surrounded by the Spanish in 1876.

Since Henry Reeve was a young U.S. internationalist, it was only fitting that the first ELAM arrivals were seven young women from the United States. They were recent graduates of ELAM who had interrupted preparations for their medical board examinations in the United States in order to live and work among the Haitian people. For them "it was no problem in sleeping in tents and working any hour of the day or night."[2]

The following week, another ELAM graduate, Marcela Vera from Colombia, arrived with a larger group of Henry Reeve volunteers. A month earlier she had tried unsuccessfully to join other relief efforts. Médecins Sans Frontières turned her down because she did not speak French, and the Red Cross told her she did not have the required two years' experience in disaster relief. When she heard that ELAM was organizing a brigade of former students, she filled up her backpack and headed to Cuba in less than forty-eight hours. Marcela and the ELAM graduates were given an intensive crash course by Havana's experts in disaster relief medicine, then sent on to Haiti to assist the experienced teams that by this time had set up more than twenty field hospitals. Once there, Marcela took up residence in a tent in a camp where the homeless were living and, like many of the ELAM arrivals, was quickly put to work vaccinating everyone against infectious diseases.[3]

In the immediate aftermath of the quake, there were a great many other foreign volunteers arriving to work on short-term assignments with various relief organizations that had no connection to Cuba. Some of them found that no one knew where they should be assigned to work, or they were sent to places where there were no supplies or coordination of any kind. But others found they could be readily incorporated into Cuban-Haitian efforts. At La Paz Hospital, one of the few medical facilities in the capital of Port-au-Prince that was not destroyed, a Cuban team had taken charge of operations the day after the earthquake. When doctors and nurses arrived from Spain, Chile, Mexico, the Dominican Republic, Canada, and other nations, they were rapidly integrated with Cuban and Haitian colleagues. Reporter Leticia Martínez Hernández described one scene: "Rosalía, a nun, was caressing a little girl whose leg was in danger due to gangrene. She came from Spain. . . . For Asmyrrehe Dollin, a Haitian doctor who graduated in Cuba, helping his compatriots is the greatest thing that life has bestowed on him. . . . Working together with the doctors who at one point were his professors, is an immense source of pride for him."[4]

Dr. Mirta Roses, the Argentine director of the Pan American Health Organization, praised the Cubans for their ability to coordinate the efforts of specialists arriving from dozens of countries: "We were already aware of their organizational capacity, their experience in disaster management; and it has been an enormous advantage that they were already here." There were well-intentioned medical volunteers, she noted, who were arriving elsewhere in Haiti without infrastructure or a work team to join; not only were their talents being wasted, but potentially they could turn into "displaced persons" themselves who would use up valuable resources that were meant to help homeless and hungry Haitians.

There were, of course, many dedicated and effective medical personnel arriving from all parts of the world who did invaluable relief work without any association with the Cuban-led contingents. But the Cubans and their ELAM-educated collaborators distinguished themselves by their ability to organize and coordinate their efforts into a long-term sustainable project. They also were the largest disaster relief presence in the country, far larger than the 269-person foreign contingent fielded by the well-funded and well-respected group Doctors Without Borders (Médecins Sans Frontières).[5]

Cuba announced that its presence was destined to become even larger about a month after the earthquake. Vice President Esteban Lazo of Cuba, after meeting with President Preval of Haiti, promised that over the long haul his nation would provide at least two thousand doctors, plus a variety of other nurses and technicians who would first devote themselves to the rehabilitation of thousands of severely injured and the prevention of epidemics. Their overall mission, however, was broader: Cuba would work with the Haitian government on the arduous long-term task of building a public health and primary care system that could serve the whole nation.

This effort was aided by Cuba's membership in the Bolivarian Alliance for the Peoples of the Americas (known by its acronym, ALBA; its other members include Bolivia, Nicaragua, Ecuador, and Venezuela). ALBA voted to concentrate a significant part of material assistance to the health system, an effort that had already begun before the quake. Five Comprehensive Diagnosis Clinics had been built with ALBA funds in different parts of the country, and five more under construction were rushed to completion by Venezuelan-Haitian work teams soon after the disaster. Venezuela, the nation that was first to send an aid shipment to Haiti the day after the quake, also canceled Haiti's debt of hundreds of millions of dollars.

Secret to Success: Lifetime Dedication

While all this assistance was being organized and delivered, the mainstream media in the United States avoided reporting on the substantive contribution of Cuba and Venezuela. However, one of the most effective U.S. providers of medical aid, Partners in Health, knew from prior firsthand experience about the expertise and value of working with Cuban medical professionals. Dr. Paul Farmer, the physician and anthropologist who was a founder of Partners in Health, has an outstanding reputation for building systems of community health care among the poor in rural Haiti and Africa. He once explained, in a 2006 interview, why his Partners in Health medical team decided they needed help from Cuban doctors even after their hospital operation in rural Haiti was well established. "We'd been here ten years working," said Farmer, "real hard work, yeoman's work, trying to deliver basic health services to poor people in central Haiti, before we asked ourselves 'Well, what have we done to beef up the public sector?' . . . It's easy in a place like Haiti for groups like ours to say 'We're doing great. We've built an OR, and we've put in a blood bank.' But you know you can always do better."

The solution? They brought in experienced specialists. Haitian doctors would have been the first choice, according to Farmer, but

Partners in Health could not find any who were interested in leaving their middle-class city lifestyles to live in the primitive countryside. So they asked Cuba for help—not for experts who would give a brief seminar on techniques that could promote public health, but for veterans who would live and work among the Partners in Health personnel. Two doctors came for the standard two-year commitment that Cuban health volunteers make when they work with their own Plan Integral de Salud medical brigades. "We asked for a pediatrician and a surgeon, and we got them," said Farmer. "The surgeon had been practicing for thirty years, all over the world. He could do anything. Any kind of emergency surgery, general surgery; he was very broadly experienced. The pediatrician had been a pediatrician for twenty-seven years. The presence of these two very mature physicians, with a lot of public health experience, really served to raise the level of care all across the hospital and the system."

The Partners in Health professionals—doctors, nurses, and health coordinators who were already known for their selfless service and willingness to live among the poor—knew they needed more on-the-job training. Cuban physician/tutors came to the rescue. As Farmer explained, "There's no substitute for that in medicine . . . for having experienced people pass on their way of delivering care to others—to trainees, to those who are younger or less experienced. But the wonderful and almost magical thing about the two of them—and about their successors—is their work ethic and their professional ethic."[6]

Transmitting Cuban Medical Skills and Ethics in Adverse Circumstances

What Dr. Paul Farmer and Partners in Health experienced on a small scale has become one of the central challenges for the Cuban medical brigades as they work in more than seventy countries around the globe. Over the course of little more than a decade, through the interplay between international medical cooperation and new kinds of medical education, Cuba has refined its ideas about how to immediately effect substantial improvements in the host nation, while at the same time transferring medical skills and ethics to the host population by allowing young people to work alongside doctors and nurses in real-life medical situations. In Haiti, which is not only terribly poor but the victim of a series of natural and political disasters, this has been especially difficult.

When the first Cuban medical brigade arrived in Haiti after Hurricane George under Plan Integral de Salud in December of 1998, at least 90 percent of Haitian doctors were practicing in the cities, even though more than two-thirds of Haitians lived in the countryside. The Cuban presence had an almost immediate medical impact: statistics for 2002 showed that the rate of infant mortality, that is, the number of babies dying at birth, was only half of what it had been just two years earlier.[7] Over the next eleven years, 6,094 Cuban medical personnel offered their assistance to the Haitian population, with anywhere from 350 to 800 working at any one time. On their two-year rotations, they gained enough expertise in communicating in Creole to spread throughout the country, espe- cially to rural areas and smaller towns, making it possible to deliver local primary care services to about three-quarters of the Haitian population. Between 1998 and 2007, they conducted almost 15 mil- lion patient visits that helped produce big changes in the overall health of the nation: the average Haitian life span increased from fifty-four to sixty-one years, and the maternity death rate, infant mor- tality rate, and the number of children dying before the age of five were all reduced by more than half. Near the end of this period, Haitian students at ELAM were returning home and beginning to assume a role in community medicine.[8]

When the first class of students from all over Latin America grad- uated from ELAM in 2005, a Haitian student, Dr. Jean Pierre Brizmar, addressed the commencement audience and spoke about his last year of internship, 2004–05, when he and other students spent six months working in the Haitian countryside. It had been a rough year, since parts of Haiti's north coast were devastated by hurricane flooding, and the whole country was shaken by political turmoil. This did not deter

Dr. Brizmar and his colleagues. "We lived with our professors," he said, referring to the Cuban doctors who supervised his internship. "And during that time, we saw 773,000 patients. We donated our own blood when necessary, and nobody went home unattended."[9]

It was remarkable that Brizmar's professors were still present in Haiti during the 2004–05 school year, because 2004 was the year the Bush administration encouraged Haiti's elite political opposition, funded through the International Republican Institute and USAID, to overthrow the government of democratically elected President Aristide. Since Aristide's government had been building even closer ties with Cuba and its medical representatives, it appeared that the new interim government of Prime Minister Gerard Latortue, in deference to Washington, would demand the departure of all 525 Cuban health workers present in the country. But it never did so, because there was no other medical alternative; the huge majority of Haitian doctors who huddled around the capital and competed for the business of well-off clients were not disposed to live in the countryside. Burnet Cherisol, director of Child Care Haiti and a former priest, described the situation after the coup: "In many areas the only care available is from the Cuban doctors, even though the current Haitian government doesn't support them. Few Haitian physicians are willing to venture out this far, where there's no electricity, no hotel. For them, the good life stops down the road."[10]

The considerable contribution of nurses and other Cuban medical professionals cannot be overlooked. They made up 40 percent of the Cuban medical personnel present in Haiti at the time of the earthquake, and in addition to providing medical care they served as important public health educators. In their spare time before the disaster, they joined Cuban literacy teams that were teaching young Haitians to read. The main beneficiaries of their instruction, however, were Haitian nurses. Cuban nurse Maritza Acosta explained to Radio Guantánamo that one important result of this training, particularly in light of the foreign aid that arrived after the quake, was that they familiarized many Haitians with the uses of modern medical technology: "We developed a program in the Diagnostic Centers with the Haitian nursing personnel, who despite being licensed and qualified, had not mastered technical elements or the modern equipment that had never arrived in the country before."[11]

The Cubans have had so much experience dealing with societies with little or no medical resources available that their own disaster relief teams come prepared for everything when they arrive on the scene. The Henry Reeve Brigade surgeons had modern operating theaters set up in tents that were functioning within forty-eight hours of their arrival in Haiti. This was because they brought their own "*electromedicos*," five-man teams of electricians who know exactly how to set up the tents in concert with sophisticated equipment powered by portable generators.

Because the Haitian disaster killed hundreds of thousands and shattered an entire society, it was also necessary to think about what would happen after emergency care was provided. In preparation for a process of recovery that would take many months and years, teams of Cuban clinical psychologists arrived to help residents work their way back from the trauma. Accompanying the psychologists was a troupe of fifty artists, musicians, dancers, puppeteers, acrobats, and clowns called the Maria Machada Brigade, who lifted spirits and provided companionship and activities for over 100,000 Haitian children and teenagers.

"First There Is God and Then the Cuban Doctors"

Observers who were familiar with Cuba's role in Haiti knew that sustained and expert aid was the key to helping Haitians create a new and viable health system. Dr. Henriette Chamouillet, who was in charge of the World Health Organization operations in Haiti after the earthquake, said that Cuban help in medical education was "absolutely" necessary. In the previous ten years, the Latin American School of Medicine in Havana had been educating as many doctors as Haiti's own national medical school, with the difference being that the Cuban-trained physicians were prepared by their educational experience to work with the poor. Dr. Chamouillet pointed out that "Cuba is training Haitian doctors, roughly 80 doctors per year. And that is for years and years and years already. Three groups of doctors, trained doctors, are already out of the university and practicing in Haiti. Most of them return to Haiti. Cuba is only keeping a few of them to train them as specialists."[12]

Dr. Patrick Dely, a Haitian who had been educated at ELAM, told reporter Conner Gorry that in the past he had seen other Haitian doctors take jobs at public hospitals that paid them very poorly. Soon they began to shift to treating patients who could pay them privately, and eventually they were only doing their hospital work one or two days a week. He thought that the same could have happened to him, except that he had been transformed during his stay in Cuba: "Like all young people, I went with my own ideas and philosophy. I had my goals and my life perspective already in place. I went to Cuba to become a doctor, to return to serve my people, of course, but also to reach a level, attain a certain lifestyle, that was beyond my previous possibilities. You know the prestige doctors enjoy in Haiti. But I hadn't been in Cuba even two years when my thinking began to change, and my goals with it."

Dr. Dely began to realize that he was already very privileged, since he had been permitted to get a good education in an honorable career, and that he didn't need any more privileges. "A new philosophy began taking shape in my mind. I began dreaming big, beyond just being a doctor for me. I started thinking about my country, and thinking about others. I started to feel a responsibility to help as many people as possible."[13]

Although the commitment of Haitians like Dr. Dely is admirable, Haiti desperately needs large-scale participation by other countries in support of the Cuban projects, so that more local health care professionals can earn adequate salaries and work in facilities equipped to treat the poor. Fortunately, the other members of ALBA, including Venezuela, had already pledged to back up the Cuban effort with their own resources. And on March 27, 2010, Haiti, Cuba, and Brazil made an important announcement about their cooperative venture that aimed to build a completely new health system. José Gomes, Brazil's Minister of Health, said his country would support the effort with $80 million plus the participation of Brazilian educators and medical personnel who would work alongside their Cuban counterparts. "Haiti needs a permanent, quality health care system," he said, "supported by well-trained professionals. . . . We will provide this, together with Cuba—a country with an extremely long internationalist experience, a great degree of technical ability, great determination, and an enormous amount of heart."

President René Preval of Haiti, who was present at the same meeting, pointed out that this project was possible because over the years the Cuban medical missions to Haiti had gained an incredible degree of trust from the local people: "For the Haitians first there is God and then the Cuban doctors. And it's not just me saying that, one who is convinced, but also poor people in the communities, the very poorest citizens."[14]

One of the ways to appreciate the special magnitude of the Cubans' role in Haiti is to compare it with the medical effort of the U.S. government immediately after the earthquake. The United States Navy was lauded, deservedly, by the U.S. media for sending the USNS *Comfort*, a hospital ship with a 550-person medical staff, and treating 871 patients and performing 843 surgical operations. But then after seven weeks, like many foreign aid providers, the ship left Haiti. During the same period of time, the Cuban medical brigades did incomparable work, attending to 227,443 patients and performing 6,499 surgeries. But that was only a small extent of their contribution because they were staying on and expanding their efforts.

By April, three months after the disaster, the Cuba/ALBA initiatives had managed to get twenty-three primary care health centers, fifteen referral hospitals, and twenty-one rehabilitation facilities "up and running" according to Cuban foreign minister Bruno Rodriguez. And this was only the beginning. At the United Nations conference on Haitian recovery, Rodriguez said that Cuba was committed "to deliver wide health coverage for the population" and listed the facilities that would be created: 101 primary health care centers, thirty community referral hospitals, thirty rehabilitation facilities, a "Haitian National Specialties Hospital," directed by eighty Cuban specialists, and new training facilities for more Haitian doctors.[15]

Clearly one of the best features of Cuban medical internationalism is that it keeps growing because it inspires others to join in. Bolivia benefited immensely from the aid provided by Cuban doctors between 2006 and 2010, and from significant investment in education and social welfare through its association with the ALBA nations. It was not surprising, then, that the La Paz newspaper *La Razon* proudly announced on February 28, 2010, that the largest foreign contingent of ELAM graduates joining the Henry Reeve Brigade in Haiti was made up of fifty young doctors from Bolivia, twenty-one women and twenty-nine men. Although almost all of these Cuban-educated doctors enjoyed medical positions and good salaries in Bolivia, they decided to leave their jobs immediately and stay for an indefinite time in Haiti; according to the paper, they would stay as long as their assistance was needed by the Haitian people. A few weeks later Dr. Lucio Pinto told reporters that he left his job in the Bolivian countryside even though he was not certain it could be held for him. "This is how to make a reality of Fidel Castro's dream when he created ELAM," he said, "going to work in the countries where doctors don't exist."

3. Creating Two, Three . . . One Hundred Thousand Che Guevaras

The life of Che is a great inspiration for every person who loves liberty.
—NELSON MANDELA, 1991

Before Che Guevara left for Bolivia in 1966, he wrote a letter to the nonaligned third world countries of Asia, Africa, and Latin America, encouraging them to unite in their efforts to escape from the historic domination of the colonialist and imperialist forces of Europe and North America. He recommended starting many revolutionary struggles and so much simultaneous resistance that the United States and its allies could not possibly subdue the forces of liberation. The letter was published the following year and the words of its title, "Create two, three . . . many Vietnams,"[1] were soon repeated around the world.

For the most part, the strategy Che recommended did not work. With the exception of Vietnam itself, and a few other nations that achieved liberation from their European masters, the third world liberation movements of the 1960s were stymied by brutal right-wing strategies or brought down by their own internal conflicts and corruption. Movements for progressive change throughout Latin America were overwhelmed by fascist military regimes that were either supported or tacitly tolerated by Washington. In the 1980s, the Reagan administration labeled Cuba a "terrorist nation" for inspiring and supporting the legitimate efforts of people fighting for freedom in Central America and Africa while the United States overtly or covertly supported an array of dictatorships, counterrevolutionary bandits, and racist regimes that wanted to destroy these liberation movements.

There was, however, another strategy still available for building international solidarity and demonstrating that "another world is possible." Between 1961 and 2008, Cuba sent 185,000 medical specialists to work in 103 nations.[2] To amplify this effort and encourage the participation of other countries, Cuba began providing a free education near the end of the 1990s for about 1,500 foreign students per year at the Latin American School of Medicine in Havana. But this would provide only a tiny fraction of the doctors the world needed.

Fidel Castro, speaking at the first graduation of doctors from ELAM in 2005, announced the solution: Cuba and Venezuela were going to join forces to educate 100,000 more doctors over the next ten years: 30,000 Venezuelans, 60,000 coming from other countries in Latin America and the Caribbean, and another 10,000 from nations in Africa and Asia. Cuba and Venezuela were committing themselves to creating a new kind of internationalist fighting force, made up of brigades battling disease and misery.

Reverberations from Bolivia

One noontime in January 2008, I was walking from our house in Monte Carmelo and passing the local Barrio Adentro clinic where nine or ten MIC medical students, dressed in their white jackets, were congregating outside. They called me over to meet their new colleagues, Karen from Peru and Georgo from Suriname, who were beginning the first-year MIC course. These two were part of a contingent of foreign students who had been selected for an experimental training program by the Latin American School of Medicine in Havana (ELAM). Rather than go to ELAM's campus in Cuba, they had come to Venezuela to join students of Medicina Integral Comunitaria at various locations around the country. According to Karen and Georgo, there were 335 foreign students in the new program, and "the really big contingent, at least half of our group, comes from Bolivia."

Bolivia? The right-wing generals thought they had knocked off Che Guevara for good in Bolivia. They assassinated him, chopped off his hands, and sent the fingerprints to Washington. They even hid his bones in an unmarked grave, where they sat undisturbed for thirty years. They thought they could kill the spirit of revolution, that there would be no more Vietnams and no more revolutionaries like Che.

Their efforts were for naught. Now there are Bolivian Dr. Guevaras, lots of them among hundreds of thousands of young idealistic people who want to follow in his footsteps, dedicated to serving humanity with a strong sense of revolutionary commitment. They were jumping at the opportunity to do exactly what the young Che wanted to do: serve the poor, heal the afflicted, make a better world.

Perhaps the CIA, which had a direct role in helping the Bolivian army capture and assassinate Che in 1967, was alarmed by this new threat forty years later. The very same week in January 2008 that foreign medical students, including Bolivians, started classes with Cuban doctors in Venezuela, the CIA presented an intelligence report to the U.S. Senate that claimed Cuba and Venezuela were having a negative effect on the governments of Bolivia, Ecuador, and Nicaragua. The Chancellor of Bolivia quickly rejected the accusations of the CIA: "I don't know where they are coming from and where they get their information. The people of Bolivia know what relations are like with Cuba and Venezuela."

What negative effect was the CIA talking about? At the time there were 2,200 Cuban health workers—1,553 doctors, plus nurses, paramedics, lab technicians, and auxiliary personnel—at work all over Bolivia, and Venezuela was financing the construction of various medical facilities. Over the previous two years, 2006 to 2008, over 300,000 Bolivians had their eyesight restored for free by Cuban doctors working in a program called Misión Milagro (Miracle Mission), which is financed by Venezuela and has provided free eye surgery to more than one and a half million people in Latin America and the Caribbean. At first, many Bolivians were flown to Cuba for surgery, and then fifteen clinics were set up in Bolivia itself under the direction of joint Cuban/Bolivian medical teams. In 2006, the Cuban ophthalmologists operated on one impoverished, anonymous man in a clinic in Santa Cruz, and shortly thereafter his son wrote the local newspaper to thank the doctors for their service to his elderly father. The man was Mario Teran, the Bolivian army sergeant who had been ordered by his superiors to murder Che Guevara after his capture in 1967.

A month after the CIA delivered its 2008 report about the evil influence of Cuba and Venezuela, ABC News ran a provocative story about Peace Corps volunteers and Fulbright scholars working on projects in Bolivia. The U.S. visitors reported that they had been appalled by the behavior of representatives from their own embassy who had approached them and asked them to spy on Cuban doctors and any other Venezuelans and Cubans who were working on aid projects.[3] For some reason, it had not occurred to the U.S. State Department that many young Americans, especially those who confronted the depth of poverty in Latin America, might not be sympathetic to the U.S. government's long-standing antipathy to the Cuban Revolution and the legacy of Che.

A few years earlier, in 2004, when Knight-Ridder reporter Kevin Hall visited the site of Guevara's death in Vallegrande and La Higuera, he encountered Emily George of North Carolina, who was making a kind of pilgrimage after finishing her Peace Corps duties in Bolivia. "Che embodied a lot of what my generation is lacking," George told him, "[in] his idealism and concern for social justice in Latin America." The degree of admiration among local people was even higher, according to farmer Manual Cortez, who lived next door to the schoolhouse in La Higuera where Guevara was murdered. "We say, 'Che, help us with our work or with this planting,' and it always goes well. He suffered almost like Our Father, in flesh and bone."[4]

Many people in the surrounding area hang pictures of Che on the walls of their houses next to images of Jesus and the Virgin Mary because they believe he brings miracles or good luck. But reporter

Nick Buxton noted in 2007 that the symbolic power of Che had taken on a powerful new earthly reality near the old hospital building in Vallegrande where Che's body (in a remarkably Christ-like pose) had been photographed by CIA agent Felix Rodriguez in 1967. Behind the hospital is a large clinic staffed by twenty-six Cuban health professionals who were providing free health care to the surrounding area. "Carmen, a Cuban nurse," wrote Buxton, "certainly felt that Che's dream was being realized. 'Just imagine if he saw this. It shows his death was not in vain.' Working seven days a week with hardly a break and far from her family, she said she gets her 'force from the Comandante.' Julio and Norma, who come from Santa Clara in Cuba, a city that Che's brigade liberated, added: 'Che said you should give yourself to others, that is what we are doing, living out the legacy of Che.'"[5]

Origin of the Cuban International Medical Brigades

Cuban revolutionaries from the very beginning felt an obligation to show "solidarity with their brothers" and go wherever in the world fellow human beings were in medical need. After the victory of the revolution in 1959, Cuba lost half of its physicians because 3,000 chose to leave the country, most of them going to the United States. Although the exodus of doctors created a severe shortage of medical personnel, some of those who remained behind were asked to volunteer for foreign missions. There were two kinds of medical brigades designed for distinctly different purposes. One dealt with immediate emergency response to relieve the suffering of people hit by natural disasters; medical personnel were expected to stay abroad for a matter of months. The other kind was meant for long-term collaboration in developing another nation's system of primary health care; the doctors and nurses who volunteered usually expected to remain for two years, at which time they would be relieved by other Cubans.

A photograph from 1960 shows Dr. Oscar Fernandez Mel, head of the Cuban College of Physicians, shaking hands with Dr. Salvador

Allende, who was a senator in the Chilean government at the time. Fernandez Mel had left urban Cuba behind in the 1950s to join the guerrillas in the Sierra Maestra, where he had provided some welcome relief to the first overburdened guerrilla/physician in Fidel's band, Dr. Guevara. In the photo, Dr. Fernandez Mel and a Cuban medical team are boarding an airplane bound from Havana to Valdivia, Chile, a small city that had just been devastated by the most powerful earthquake that has ever been recorded anywhere in the world. The first Cuban disaster relief brigade was flying to the aid of the injured and homeless.

Cuban disaster relief brigades will serve in any country, regardless of its political or religious orientation, and in some cases have helped nations with which Cuba had no diplomatic relations. For example, in 1972 Nicaragua was still under the firm dictatorial grip of the notoriously corrupt Somoza family, which not only had mistreated its own population but had openly allowed the CIA to train Cuban exiles in their territory for the Bay of Pigs invasion of 1961. Nevertheless, when an earthquake flattened almost all of the capital city of Managua, Cuba rushed a disaster relief brigade to the scene.

The other kind of Cuban medical aid, concentrating on long-term medical assistance, was given to Algeria in 1963. This was a gesture of Cuban solidarity with the revolutionary government of Prime Minister Ben Bella immediately after the Algerian National Liberation Front had concluded its long anticolonial war against the French. Within a week of their arrival, a group of fifty-eight Cuban medical professionals began to fill some of the gaps in health care delivery that had been created by the rapid departure of French doctors.

One of the Cuban volunteers was Dr. Sara Perelló, who was born in 1920 and had begun a career in fine art before taking up medical studies in Havana, where she graduated in 1953. When she was interviewed in 2004 by journalist Hedelberto Lopez Blanch, Dr. Perelló was pleased to point out that 1953 was the same year Che Guevara received his medical degree in Buenos Aires. In 1963, when she was employed as a specialist in pediatric medicine at a Havana hospital, she and her mother were listening to a radio program about Ben Bella of Algeria and his revolutionary solidarity with Cuba. Her mother turned to her and said, *"Hay que ayudar a este muchacho"* (We ought to help this boy)." Because Dr. Perelló's husband encouraged her and reassured her that her aging mother would be well cared for, she immediately volunteered to join the medical brigade that was leaving for Algeria.

Forty years later, Dr. Perelló could still recount many details about delivering medical assistance in Algeria and her friendly relationships with Algerian families. She reflected upon the impact the mission had on her and her colleagues: "For us, as doctors, it made us grow as humans. It let us see the role that doctors really ought to have, since the majority of us were educated under capitalism, with lessons and concepts very distant from those proposed by the Revolution." She said the Cuban doctors had become more useful in their profession, for it was endowed with a higher purpose. The indefatigable Perelló never lost that sense of purpose; in 2004, at the age of eighty-four, she was still teaching a course on "The Mitigation of Disasters" at a medical school in Havana.[6]

Cuba's Unprecedented Role in Africa

After Algeria, and throughout five decades, Cuba devoted many missions of international solidarity to Africa, with more than half a million Cuban volunteers participating. Cuba's biggest commitment by far was in aid to Angola immediately after it won its war of independence against Portugal. When South Africa began attacking Angola, Mozambique, and Namibia and backing mercenary armies (with the assistance of the CIA) in 1975, Cuba insisted on aiding the government of the MPLA (People's Liberation Movement of Angola), even though the Soviet Union was reluctant to give armed support to African revolutionary movements. While Washington accused Cuba of exporting revolution, the Cubans pointed out that they were defending a liberation movement and revolution that had already succeeded but was now threatened by extremely reactionary forces, in particular the apartheid regime in South Africa. Thousands of doctors, nurses, medical technicians, and other civilian experts assisted Angola's revolutionary government, but they were not nearly as numerous as the 300,000 Cuban soldiers who rotated through tours of duty over the next sixteen years. Cuban troops finally left Angola in May 1991, right after the peace agreement went into effect that would assure the end of threats from South Africa. Over a sixteen-year period in Angola, there were more than 10,000 Cuban casualties, and 2,077 soldiers lost their lives. The Cuban presence not only fortified Angola, it helped liberate the continent.

Two months after the last Cubans returned home, on July 26, 1991, Nelson Mandela, who had been elected president of South Africa the previous year, visited Cuba to thank the nation. "The people of Cuba hold a very special place in the hearts of the African people," he said. "In the history of Africa there is no other case of a people that has risen up in our defense." In 1995, at the first meeting of Southern Africans in Solidarity with Cuba, he repeated the message: "Cubans came to our region as doctors, teachers, soldiers, agricultural experts, but never as colonizers. They have shared the same trenches with us in the struggle against colonialism, underdevelopment, and apartheid."[7]

Since 1991 Cuba's international aid to Africa has been strictly nonmilitary. When South Africa came under the democratic rule of the African majority, it began asking Cuba for assistance in dealing with staggering medical problems, such as devising programs to fight the extraordinarily high rate of HIV infection and helping to alleviate the shortage of physicians in impoverished rural areas. At times, as many as four hundred Cuban doctors worked in underserved areas, even though they were often criticized by South African physicians for intruding in the country's medical system. In reality, South Africa had two medical systems, an expensive European-style, for-profit system that for the most part served the white population, and a barely functioning public system that was supposed to serve the impoverished African majority. In the poorest province, the Eastern Cape, where there is a critical shortage of general practitioners, thirty-two Cuban specialists joined the faculty of the Walter Sisulu Medical School in order to help correct the problem. But South Africa, which is as rich in natural resources as Venezuela, is not politically prepared to redistribute the wealth of the country and generate a massive reallocation of medical and social resources.

On the other hand, South Africa and other relatively richer African countries such as Nigeria and Angola did pledge to use modest amounts of income from natural resources to help some of the most desperate nations on the continent. At the Group of 77 meeting of 2000, attended by many developing countries, they decided to provide funds to pay the salaries of 3,000 Cuban doctors who would serve the poorest countries by developing new infrastructures for primary health care and education.[8] Even though 777 African students continued to study medicine in Cuba between 2005 and 2009, the Cubans had already begun to shift the bulk of their attention to the African continent, where they were developing new medical education programs for physicians and other health professionals in Guinea Bissau, Equatorial Guinea, and Gambia.

These efforts began at the same time that Cuban educators were reevaluating the medical curriculum used for both their own and foreign students within Cuba. Dr. Yiliam Jimenez, a physician and Cuba's Vice Minister of Foreign Relations for International Cooperation, explained the need for changes in training methods to an international aid conference in 2008: "Traditional models of medical training cannot resolve the terrible lack of health professionals and the urgent need for access to health care in today's world." For this reason, Cuba had revised its own highly acclaimed medical education programs to establish new medical schools *extra muros*, that is, "outside the walls" of traditional universities. This was not only happening in Cuba and on a grand scale in Venezuela, but in smaller new programs being set up in Bolivia and Africa. "We are returning to the tutorial method," said Dr. Jimenez, "supplemented by information technologies and other teaching aids, so that students from low-income families can be educated in classrooms and clinics in their own communities, where their services are so sorely needed."[9]

In 2009, I chatted with journalist Hedelberto Lopez Blanch who, when he is not writing incisive articles for the Cuban press on the global political economy, is turning out short books about the missions of Cuban medical professionals abroad, for instance, *Historias Secretas De Medicos Cubanos* (Secret Stories of Cuban Doctors), which recounts testimonies of physicians who went on clandestine missions with African guerrilla armies in the 1960s and '70s. Lopez Blanch had just returned from visiting one of the latest missions of Cuban doctors in Africa, a brand- new medical school in Zanzibar, the island in the Indian Ocean that forms part of Tanzania. In 2007, Cuban medical educators went there to prepare the launch of the first Programa de Formación de Médicos para la Comunidad (Program of Medical Education for the Community) in Africa. The Zanzibar medical school was established along the same lines as the six-year programs that are currently preparing tens of thousands of physicians in Cuba and Venezuela to practice comprehensive community medicine. The forty students who made up the first class in 2008 included twenty men and twenty women, and the latter, in keeping with their own local communities, wore traditional Muslim dress. All of them spoke very good Spanish, according to Lopez Blanch, because they had completed eight months of intensive classes and needed to be able to converse with their professors. Like the students being prepared by professor/tutors in other Cuban medical education programs, the Zanzibar group split their time between working alongside their professors at local medical facilities and attending formal classes.[10]

Cuba and Disaster Relief: Kashmir, Pakistan

In addition to its great commitment to long-term medical assistance and education programs abroad, Cuba continues to expand the strength of its highly trained international disaster relief teams. This buildup gained international attention in the fall of 2005, when over 1,500 medical personnel trained in disaster medicine, the Henry Reeve Brigade, were gathered at the Havana airport with first-aid packs on their backs, ready to fly to the U.S. Gulf Coast and aid the victims of the horrendous flooding caused by Hurricane Katrina.

The Bush administration immediately rejected the offer from Havana, dismissing the humanitarian gesture as an empty propaganda ploy. The Cubans would soon demonstrate this was not the case. Only a month after Hurricane Katrina hit the United States, the Henry Reeve Brigade, all 1,536 members, was dispatched to the mountains of Kashmir in Pakistan after an enormous earthquake killed thousands of people and left hundreds of thousands homeless just as the harsh winter season was about to begin. Various other international relief groups also arrived with aid, including European and U.S. teams that each set up large base camps and stayed for a month. The Cubans stayed for seven months, building seven major base camps and thirty-two field hospitals as their medical force was augmented to include over 2,400 volunteers. The Cubans, who had never seen real winter before, not only weathered severe temperatures, but had to survive tents collapsing in the snow when their field hosptitals were snow-bound for a week after a blizzard. Before they departed, they trained 450 Pakistani doctors in the procedures necessary to operate the equipment and field hospitals they left behind.

Bruno Rodríguez, who became Cuban Foreign Minister in 2009, was Deputy Foreign Minister when he arrived in Pakistan in 2005 with the Henry Reeve Brigade. He spent the next seven months helping with the relief effort, which eventually led to the two countries establishing formal diplomatic relations for the first time since 1990. Before he left Pakistan, it was announced that one thousand Pakistani students would be given free scholarships to attend medical school in Cuba.

Difficulties Encountered in Promoting Cuban Medical Aid:
Honduras and Guatemala

Honduras and Guatemala were two of the first countries to send students to the Latin American School of Medicine in Havana in 1998. Although several hundred students from these countries were pro-gressing well in their course work over the next five years, it became apparent that there would have to be improvements in Cuba's relations with their home countries if they were going to effectively serve their fellow citizens upon their return.

In 2004, during a severe dengue fever epidemic in Tegucigalpa, the capital of Honduras, more than 400 Honduran medical students left their studies at the ELAM to join health brigades of Cuban doctors to help control the outbreak. The students treated the sick and educated the public about prevention measures. Many of them would be part of the first graduating class at ELAM the following year and they hoped to get further training in residencies working alongside the Cubans serving in their country. Unfortunately, 2005 was the year that conservative president Maduro of Honduras, prodded by the Honduran Medical Association, announced that the brigade of Cuban doctors was going to be expelled because their presence was disruptive. The medical association claimed that the Cubans were putting local doctors out of work, when in reality, as in other countries, few Honduran doctors were interested in caring for poor people in isolated areas of the country. Right-wing pressure from the likes of columnist Mary McGrady of the *Wall Street Journal* stoked an atmosphere of antipathy among the Honduran elite and their foreign allies; McGrady wrote that the doctors were "Fidel's foot soldiers" who had "the potential for soft indoctrination, a kind of tilling the soil in the poor countryside so that it is ready when political opportunity presents itself, as it has in Venezuela of late."

Unexpectedly, there was so much protest in favor of the Cuban presence by ordinary members of civil society, labor unions, and community organizations throughout Honduras that the president had to rescind the order.[11] Just a few months later, Maduro was replaced by a new, moderately liberal president, José Manuel Zelaya Rosales, who rapidly befriended the Cuban and Venezuelan governments and pledged considerable support to Honduran medical students coming home. When ELAM graduates returned to the Garifuna region on the Honduran Mosquitia Coast in 2005 and 2006, they were slated to get postgraduate residency training from Cuban specialists and a handful of Honduran doctors who opted to participate. This enabled some graduates to serve their own people in new hospital facilities such as the facility constructed in the isolated town of Ciriboya with help from progressive labor unions and not-for-profit U.S. sources of medical equipment. In 2008, the new buildings were dedicated by President Zelaya in a ceremony attended by the Cuban health representatives and the engineers who helped design and equip the facility. In a startling change of heart, representatives from the Honduran Medical Association, which three years earlier was trying to chase the Cuban doctors out of the country, joined the celebration.[12]

Unfortunately, this recognition of the value of the Cuban partnership lasted only briefly, until the summer of 2009, when the Honduran oligarchy and military, with the help of Cuban exiles in Miami, engineered a coup against President Zelaya. In the aftermath, soldiers harassed medical staff and threatened to close down the Garifuna hospital. The founder of the hospital, Dr. Luther Castillo, who had been the first Garifuna to graduate from ELAM, had to go into hiding to escape persecution and was forced to abandon the country. In 2010, he served as the coordinator of the first large contingent of ELAM graduates in the Henry Reeve Brigade when they rushed to Haiti to serve as medical volunteers after the earthquake.

In Guatemala, the Cuban presence also provoked controversy and considerable opposition from right-wing elements. In the year 2000, the "Secret Anti-Communist Army" (ESA) sent letters that threatened the lives of the 459 Cuban doctors and medical personnel working in the country. The ESA letters, published in the daily newspaper *Siglo XXI*, accused the Cubans of being "mercenaries cloaked in the noble medical profession" who were spreading "totalitarian communist ideas." And they warned: "If they do not immediately abandon the country, the executions will begin." The Guatemalan government never reacted to the threat, and the Cubans never budged.

The medical brigades have stayed on for another decade as fresh Cuban volunteers keep replacing those who finish their tours of duty. Furthermore, the political climate became more favorable, not just toward the Cubans but also toward the young people who had been educated in Cuba. In Guatemala, when President Colom took office in January of 2008, he immediately dispatched his newly elected vice president, Dr. Rafael Espada, on an official trip to Cuba to study the Cuban health system. Dr. Espada, an experienced cardiologist who once trained and worked in the United States, visited the 900 Guatemalan medical students who were studying at ELAM and praised the quality of their education.[13] By the end of 2008, the support of President Colom and Dr. Espada was proving advantageous to many graduates who could now return home to postgraduate training approved by the Guatemalan medical association. In 2009 and 2010, these former students were able to complete their residencies by working alongside Cuban professors in community medicine at rural Guatemalan clinics, or they could join other Cuban doctors who came to help train ELAM graduates in the specialties the Guatemalan health ministry had determined were most necessary. For the first time, Cuban doctors were invited to work alongside Guatemalan experts in five hospitals, training new specialists in pediatrics, orthopedics, anesthesiology, gynecology/obstetrics, and surgery.

4. Medicine in Revolutionary Cuba

Often we need to change our concepts, not only the general concepts, the social or philosophical ones, but also sometimes our medical concepts.

— CHE GUEVARA, "On Revolutionary Medicine," 1960

No other country has been as consistent in taking measures towards achieving the goal of "Health for All" as Cuba.

— DR. HALFDAN MAHLER, former director of the World Health Organization, 2000

Cuba's extraordinary ability to deliver health care and build new medical systems, in cooperation with Venezuela and other nations, was developed over a period of decades. To comprehend how a relatively small and poor country managed to make this commitment, it is necessary to understand how Cuba's human resources, scientific knowledge, and social expertise were developed in the course of building its own medical system. Immediately after the triumph of the Revolution in 1959, Cuba made changes in the ways it delivered medical services and began to emphasize preventive care. With time, they also revamped the training of health professionals to promote the comprehensive integration of family health care in community life. Although

Cuba never wavered in its desire to build a first-class health system, it had to be designed and constructed within the limited parameters of a developing country that was often operating in very difficult economic circumstances. This required a willingness to experiment while still maintaining an unwavering philosophical commitment to providing universal care. Since Cuba succeeded in building a unique health care system that serves all of its people, it became especially qualified to deliver appropriate aid and training to the poorest nations of the world.

Cuba's egalitarian medical system is the envy of most developing countries, and many developed nations as well. Its medical performance, as measured by global statistical standards such as infant and child mortality rates and adult longevity, bears this out, as does an educational system that has been able to produce more physicians per capita than any other nation on earth. By 2009, Cuba had 74,880 physicians, or one doctor for every 150 citizens, compared to one for every 330 in Western Europe, and one for every 417 in the United States.[1]

In 1958, before the Revolution, there were over 6,000 doctors in Cuba, or one for every 1,051 people, a ratio somewhat higher than most other Latin American countries. This ratio deteriorated quickly, as many physicians decided they did not want to practice medicine in a revolutionary society and left Cuba to seek their fortunes elsewhere. By the mid-1960s, only half, 3,000, remained, and the process of rebuilding their ranks was by necessity slow. When the University of Havana Medical School reopened in 1959 (the dictator Batista had closed the university in 1956), only twenty-three of its 161 medical professors returned to teach.[2]

Despite this handicap, the revolutionary government insisted on trying to provide health care for all Cubans as quickly as possible. It absorbed all private insurance programs, health care services, and hospitals into a national public system. Prices for medicines were reduced and pharmaceutical companies were quickly nationalized. Fees for treatment were gradually reduced and ultimately eliminated. An effort to mobilize care for the entire population caused considerable commotion at the University of Havana Medical School in 1959.

Students who were finishing their last year of study held "a series of stormy meetings"[3] and argued about whether they should be obligated to work in internships that served those who had been deprived of health care in the past. Many wanted to stay in the cities and train for traditional practices, but the majority decided to volunteer to go to regions of the Cuban countryside where campesinos had never received medical attention. The Ministry of Public Health followed up by creating 318 new positions for graduating doctors in the Rural Health Service, mostly in remote mountainous areas such as the Sierra Maestra. This effort was to serve as a model for all new doctors in the future, so that by the late 1960s all graduates were required to work within a public health system that provided free services to all.

The following year, when Che Guevara gave his talk "On Revolutionary Medicine," he reflected upon the situation of those medical graduates who were reluctant to serve voluntarily in rural areas. Rather than simply criticize that group for its lack of solidarity with the Revolution and the poor, Che chose to emphasize that their reluctance was due to something more than greed and acknowledged that he, as a medical student, had idealistic dreams of individual glory but was not yet prepared for a life of revolutionary solidarity:

A few months ago, here in Havana, it happened that a group of newly graduated doctors did not want to go into the country's rural areas and demanded remuneration before they would agree to go. From the point of view of the past it is the most logical thing in the world for this to occur; at least, so it seems to me, for I can understand it perfectly. The situation brings back to me the memory of what I was and what I thought a few years ago. . . .

When I began to study medicine, the majority of the concepts I have today, as a revolutionary, were absent from my store of ideals. Like everyone, I wanted to succeed. I dreamed of becoming a famous medical research scientist; I dreamed of working indefatigably to discover something which would be used to help humanity, but which signified a personal triumph for me. I was, as we all are, a child of my environment.

Che was acknowledging that the idealistic dreams of individual glory did not necessarily prepare students for a life of social solidarity, so it was not surprising that some young doctors could not make a commitment to the revolution, even though they were living in the midst of it. As those students left the island along with other experienced physicians, Cuba had to begin educating their replacements with just one medical school at the University of Havana. Che's old friend Alberto Granado, the Argentine who had accompanied him on his motorcycle journey around South America, helped remedy the situation. Granado, who had earned degrees in biochemistry and dedicated himself to work on leprosy, moved to Cuba in 1960 to support the Revolution. By 1962, he and a group of Cuban doctors opened the second medical university in the country, located in Santiago de Cuba, 500 miles from Havana. Although it began with only sixty-three students, forty-five years later it had grown to include 18,333 students in five schools, two for medicine, and one each for nursing, dentistry, and allied health sciences. As of 2008, there were twenty-five medical schools in Cuba, and 29,000 Cuban students of medicine, who were just a small fraction of the 202,000 students enrolled in all medical fields, among them dentistry, nursing, medical technology, and rehabilitation.

Still, it took until 1976 for the country to regain its prerevolutionary ratio of doctors to citizens. Even though the percentage of physicians was no higher than in 1958, the Cuban health delivery system had achieved exceptional gains in terms of reducing mortality, because the doctors and other medical workers were now deployed in an entirely different manner. The new national health service attempted to provide doctors for all underserved areas; it emphasized various preventive measures in public health programs that could reach all citizens; and it created high awareness of health issues among the general public because of government education campaigns that involved volunteers in every neighborhood.

When doctors who had gone to the mountains as part of the first wave of the Rural Medical Service in the 1960s were interviewed many years later, they looked back at their experience as a major factor in preparing them to practice a new kind of medicine. The interviewers noted a common progression of their experience: at first "doctors lived in people's huts" and "their role was solely to care for the sick, given the huge number of patients who came to see them daily." Then, over time, "as the doctors became more integrated into the communities, their social and educational role came into its own."[4] Many of these doctors went on to be leading figures in Cuban medicine over the decades that followed; their early experience of living among the poor and learning about the sources of their illnesses had laid the moral groundwork for the universal emphasis on preventive and primary care.

In the 1970s, local polyclinics were established and became the core institutions for providing comprehensive community care with an emphasis on primary care delivered efficiently to the whole population. In order to make doctors, nurses, and other health care professionals more cognizant of their obligation to create healthy communities, oversight of all medical education was transferred from the Ministry of Education to the Ministry of Public Health in 1976. The Ministry of Public Health recommended immediate changes:

> Traditionally our doctors have been educated almost exclusively in the hospital, with a clear tendency to turn themselves into technicians of diseases, and without sufficient training in the sociological, psychological, or hygienic-epidemiological aspects of health. . . . Primary attention was undervalued. . . . For decades there was an exaggerated tendency toward specialization . . . that has deformed the conception of the human.[5]

To make the polyclinic model function as a hub for primary care, it would be necessary to change the paradigms of medical education and health care philosophy over the coming decades. When Cuban medical experts refer to the history of the advances they have made, they nearly always refer to the guidelines laid down at Alma-Ata in 1978, when an International Conference on Primary Health Care was held in that city in the Soviet Union (now in present-day Kazakhstan). The conclusions of the conference, issued in a report by the World Health Organization and the United Nations Children's Fund, set an international agenda for developing universal health in all nations, and particularly the developing world. The report emphasized new health delivery systems built around the primacy of primary care, with family practitioners trained to integrate medical treatment with public health initiatives and preventive education.[6] Immediately after the conference, there was great enthusiasm for this idea among health experts and medical schools in many parts of the world, including developed countries like the United States and Canada that have vast rural areas and impoverished urban centers with severe shortages of medical personnel.

But over the next couple of decades the push to redesign medical education to prioritize primary care health delivery waned throughout much of the world, both in capitalist systems captivated by the profits to be made in "health care markets" and in developing economies decimated by neoliberal policies that could not contemplate investing in public health services. Dr. Halfdan Mahler of Denmark, director of the World Health Organization (WHO) from 1973 to 1988, reflected on the meaning of Alma-Ata Declaration in 2008: "For most, it was a true revolution in thinking. 'Health for all' is a value system with primary health care as the strategic component. The two go together." He suggested that the global consensus on emphasizing public health and primary care had been achieved because "the 1970s was a warm decade for social justice. That's why, after Alma-Ata in 1978, everything seemed possible." Likewise, when the idea of comprehensive health care based on social equity was rapidly abandoned in most parts of the world in the following decade, it was because of "an abrupt reversal, when the International Monetary Fund (IMF) promoted the Structural Adjustment Program with all kinds of privatization, and that drew skepticism toward the Alma-Ata consensus and weakened commitment to the primary health care strategy. WHO regions kept on fighting in countries, but there was no support from the World Bank and the IMF."[7]

Cuba, however, remained devoted to the Alma-Ata vision and added new features to its own health care system every decade to make that vision become a reality. In the 1980s, the Ministry of Public Health was able to provide for the training of more qualified primary health specialists because medical school faculties were created in every province of the country. By 1984, Fidel Castro announced that Cuba would have 75,000 doctors by the year 2000, creating such a surplus that it would allow for 10,000 of them to serve overseas at any one time. In 1986, in the interests of accuracy, the government adjusted this goal to 65,000 physicians, a number that was surpassed by the turn of the century, when there were 66,000 doctors, an astounding change, from one doctor for every 1,000 people in 1976 to one per 167 twenty-four years later.

In 1984, the Ministry of Public Health also took a step toward making all these future doctors suitable for primary health promotion. It adopted a program of family medicine called *medicina general integral*, which is usually referred to as "comprehensive general medicine" in English. By the end of the decade, this program was graduating specialists in comprehensive general medicine and creating Basic Health Teams, composed of one doctor and one nurse, that were assigned to serve every small neighborhood in the country throughout the 1990s. These teams were assisted by *brigadistas sanitarias*, health brigades made up of neighborhood residents, who met frequently with the doctors and nurses and were especially valuable in promoting preventive care and participation in public health campaigns.

By 2004, the teams were able to serve more than 99 percent of all Cubans, with each team having a small urban neighborhood or a rural area composed of 120 to 150 families (about 700 to 800 individuals) under their care. The doctor and nurse were generally required to live in the neighborhood they served, readily available for visits to each family; this was key to the practice of preventive medicine because it allowed the team to understand the most pressing medical issues of their neighborhood. By gathering vital statistics on everyone, and then emphasizing preventive care and health education, the doctors and nurses made Cuban citizens more conscious of maintaining good health, which led to a marked reduction in hospitalization rates. The doctor/nurse teams could refer patients to the diagnostic centers at the

polyclinics for laboratory testing and examination by medical specialists, and they, in turn, could send patients to hospitals for treatment or
surgery when necessary. Each polyclinic was located where it could
serve a sizable cluster of doctor/nurse teams and anywhere from
20,000 to 40,000 people.

When a team of family medicine experts from the United States
reviewed the primary care accomplishments of Cuba in the early
1990s, they emphasized the incredible thoroughness of the attention
given by doctor and nurse teams, who literally knew everyone in their
assigned areas. "Each family practitioner," they wrote, "is required to
see every patient in his or her catchment area at least twice a year. The
physician maintains a record of preventive services and conditions for
all patients in the catchment area." They described things that would
strike the U.S. medical consumer as unbelievable: "The family physician travels personally to the referral hospital. There, he or she meets
with specialists who assume responsibility for the patient's inpatient
management, coordinates inpatient services to assure continuity after
discharge, and maintains frequent contacts with the patient to
enhance the long-term patient-doctor relationship."[8]

With the proliferation of the family doctor-and-nurse program, the
general medical curriculum was changed to fit the family doctor
model. In the 1990s it was decided that almost all medical students
should be trained first in family medicine, including a three-year residency, before moving on to other specialties.

Besides guaranteeing the primacy of family/community care
within Cuba, this insistence on competency at the primary level gave
the Cuban volunteers a great deal of flexibility for future medical missions to countries with severe deficits of health providers. All doctors
were capable of providing consistent comprehensive family care, but
those who completed other specialty degrees, and there were many of
these, could offer other kinds of medical expertise when necessary.

Dr. Ileana del Rosario Morales Suárez, Dr. José A. Fernández
Sacasas, and Dr. Francisco Durán García outlined the changing concepts for medical education that were instituted at that time. In
making all physicians competent in primary health delivery, these key

elements were emphasized: 1) medicine is conceived as a sociobiological science integrated with real-life processes; 2) problem-based and interactive learning methods are used to increase cognitive independence; 3) more epidemiology and public health science are emphasized; 4) medical and clinical skills are introduced earlier in the training; 5) professors are asked to keep improving their teaching methods and students are asked to participate in service learning; 6) all medical schools are required to have departments of comprehensive general medicine; and 7) before students take their theoretical exams, they must pass a practical exam that shows mastery of skills and procedures that are needed for family medicine.[9]

Health Care during the Special Period

Since the Cuban economy grew at a brisk annual rate of about 4 percent from 1975 to 1989, conditions seemed ideal for the nation to keep expanding the primary care system with the doctor and nurse teams, as well as implementing the new medical training program in *medicina general integral.* Unfortunately, 1989 was the year major changes in the international political economy would force Cuba to live through the "Special Period," the very difficult decade that threatened not only the survival of its health system but the revolution itself.

With the collapse of Cuba's trading partners in the Soviet Union and Eastern Europe at the beginning of the 1990s, Cuba suffered a 76 percent decline in exports, and within four years, 1989 to 1993, the nation's Gross Domestic Product fell by 35 percent. The population had to adjust to drastic changes in lifestyle, such as the shortage of fuel that required many Cubans to travel on bikes and horse-drawn carriages instead of in cars and buses, and use oxen for plowing fields instead of tractors. Food shortages became so serious by 1993 and 1994 that the average calorie intake fell, especially among adult men where it declined by at least 25 percent. Only the strict rationing of food made it possible to feed nursing mothers and the infirm their prescribed diets while providing young children with their daily milk rations and 100 percent of the necessary calories.

The U.S. Congress was determined to make things even worse for Cuba by enacting the Torrecelli law, the ignominiously named Cuba Democracy Act, in 1992. With the intention of hastening the total collapse of Cuban society, the law ordered U.S. corporations with subsidiaries in other countries to stop all commerce with Cuba and with foreign companies that traded with Cuba. Because food, medicines, and medical supplies represented 90 percent of Cuban trade with U.S. subsidiaries as of 1992, the Torrecelli law exacerbated medication shortages that were already affecting Cuban patients. As the Special Period became more severe during 1993 and 1994, about half of 1,200 commonly used medicines were unavailable at local pharmacies; this meant increased human suffering—for example, hundreds of thousands of asthmatics were without necessary medication. In 1993 the dietary deprivation was so extreme that more than 50,000 Cubans suffered an epidemic of optic neuropathy, a serious affliction of the eyes and nervous system that was probably caused by a deficiency of vitamin B complex.[10] Generally there was a shortage of antibiotics, equipment, current textbooks, and basic medical supplies; for example, the number of X rays declined by 75 percent because of a shortage of X ray film and replacement parts for broken machines.

In the face of this crisis, the Cuban government continued to devote resources to primary health care and proceeded with plans to increase the number of family doctors, even though the nation was so strapped for money it could not even afford to print new textbooks for the burgeoning group of students in comprehensive general medicine. During the decade of the 1990s, four times more doctors had been educated than in the 1970s; in 1985 there had been 10,000 family doctors practicing in the whole country; by the year 2000, their ranks had tripled to 31,000 who served alongside a similar number of nurses. Foreign medical experts were of the opinion that Cuba had avoided a "human catastrophe" during the Special Period and attributed this to the rapid expansion of the new system of Basic Health Teams delivering comprehensive and preventive care at the neighborhood level. After a brief dip in statistical health indicators for two years in the mid-90s, mortality rates decreased through the rest of the decade and showed an overall improvement compared to the figures of the 1980s.

In addition to expanded primary care, other developments began to change the conception of "good health" in Cuba during the Special Period. Hospitals encouraged new mothers to stay in the hospital longer and enjoy the benefit of a better diet at the same time that they promoted breast-feeding: the prevalence of breast-feeding at the time of discharge rose from 63 percent in 1990 to 97 percent in 1994. Although the average diet for most people was deficient in protein due to the shortages of meat, there was a healthy side to the equation: people were consuming less fat. As production of food became more local due to shortages of fuel and chemical fertilizers, small-scale urban cooperatives began producing organic food and Cubans began consuming a healthier mixture of fruits and vegetables. In many places, such as Havana, the growth of the *organiponicos,* the organic community gardens, were encouraged after the Special Period, and now provide most of the produce consumed in the city.

An emerging interest in alternative medicine and folk healing methods, including the use of herbal remedies, was accelerated during the Special Period because of an interest in finding substitutes for the allopathic pharmaceuticals that were in short supply. By the second half of the 1990s, the Ministry of Public Health distributed guidelines compiled by a panel of scientists concerning *medicina verde,* or "green medicine," based on the use of medicinal plants. Most hospitals and clinics prominently posted lists of recommended herbal treatments and the conditions, ranging from gastritis to muscle pain, that they might remedy. This increasing respect for alternative medicine had a lasting effect on Cuban medicine, for it was incorporated as a regular part of the curriculum of all the medical schools in Cuba and came to include curative measures from other cultures, such as acupuncture.

In 2000, as Cuba gradually emerged from the shadow of the Special Period, its health system was worn and tired but still intact. The United Nations Development Program published a study on human development and equity that stated: "An evaluation of 25 countries in the Americas, measuring relative inequalities in health, revealed that Cuba is the country with the best health situation in Latin America and the Caribbean. It is also the country which has achieved the most effective impact with resources, although scarce, invested in the health sector."[11]

When two Cuban medical professors, Dr. Clarivel Presno Labrador and Dr. Felix Sansó Soberat, wrote about the development of the family medical program in 2004, they praised the positive overall impact of the program and the measures that had been taken to save the health care system during the Special Period, but they also pointed out that the hardships had taken a toll on many health care professionals. One of the lasting effects was the psychological stress suffered because "family doctors and nurses, living in the communities they served, witnessed daily the harsh effects of the economic crisis on their patients, sharing their difficulties and the effects on their health." As the Cuban economy had continued to improve in the new century, they wrote, it was extremely important that the Cuban government and the Ministry of Health had decided to initiate a new effort, "a revolution within the revolution," with the express purpose of "increasing accessibility to health services by bringing them still closer to the population as a whole, and improving the all-around quality of medical care."[12]

Rebuilding Cuba's Medical System

As the twenty-first century began, Cuba was poised to integrate a variety of innovative ideas into its various medical training programs, both at home and abroad. A new curriculum was developed that made use of technological innovations and integrated the biomedical sciences into a more coherent relationship with medical practice. Dr. Juan Carrizo, dean of the Latin American School of Medicine, explained why the changes in curriculum benefit the foreign students who come to ELAM:

We have replaced the teaching of sciences in isolation—anatomy one semester, microbiology the next—with a morphophysiological pedagogical approach, which enables students to better analyze, problem-solve and integrate knowledge in a cumulative, comprehensive way. We design our courses so that everything is connected, making it easier to understand the patient as a whole, while being careful not to compromise the quality of the students' scientific training. We have found that students absorb scientific knowledge better with this methodology and are better prepared to solve clinical health problems, pursue research and develop professionally.[13]

This kind of curriculum and training was developed not only for ELAM students but for all medical students studying in Cuba. As of 2008, there were 17,000 Cuban students at the twenty-one traditional medical faculties in the various provinces, and there were another 12,000 Cubans taking advantage of a new kind of medical education that had been created outside the walls of traditional schools in 2004–05, called the University Polyclinic Medical Training Program (Programa de Medicina Polyclinica Universitaria). This program utilizes 292 of the country's 498 polyclinics, with all formal classes taking place within classrooms at each polyclinic. Most of the extensive practical training involves caring for patients alongside physicians at community primary care facilities connected to a particular polyclinic and also includes experience in the clinic's laboratory, rehabilitation facilities, and documentation center. A lesser amount of practical training, about 20 percent, takes place in hospitals and other facilities.

Finally, a variation on the polyclinic model was also utilized in 2007–08 for instituting a new physician training program for another 14,000 international students (above and beyond the 10,000 at ELAM). The New Program for the Training of Latin American Doctors (El Nuevo Programa de Formacion de Medicos Latinoamericanos, or NPFML) is training students from thirty-six countries, including the 1,000 from Pakistan who were granted free scholarships after the Cuban relief effort in Kashmir in 2005–06. Students graduating from the new program will receive diplomas as medical doctors from ELAM, even though they are being educated in other parts of the country. Groups of polyclinics were chosen as the teaching centers in four distinct "polos" under the direction of medical faculties of four different Cuban provinces: Pinar del Rio in the west, Matanzas and Cienfuegos in the central part of the country, and Holguin in the east.

Aside from making advances in the medical curriculum, Cuba was able to rebuild various parts of the health care system that had suffered from the economic devastation of the Special Period. Major investments were made to repair neglected polyclinics and hospitals and acquire technological systems that were adequate to the high degree of scientific competency that doctors, nurses, and technicians had obtained over the years. Dr. Cristina Luna, the national director of ambulatory care, has stressed that the medical system relies more and more on the polyclinics as the organizing centers of most Cuban health care: "Since 2007, the polyclinics are expected to play a leading role among all health-related institutions in their communities," thus incorporating directors and experts from homes for the elderly, pharmacies, maternity centers, and other local health institutions into a cohesive team.

The major new role of the revamped polyclinics in creating more health professionals comes at a time when the number of Cuban physicians living and working all over the world is approaching 20,000, far exceeding Fidel's ambitious goal that was set in the mid-1980s. Not only do continuing commitments abroad demand a steady stream of medical volunteers, but according to Dr. Luna, there is another absolute priority: the primary care system needs many more doctors, "42 percent more, to make sure we have enough to meet all our commitments to our own people."[14]

As the role of the polyclinic has been redefined, the public has had to make some changes, too, and not all of them have been easy. The number of people served by the old doctor-nurse teams was small enough that the family doctor seemed almost "like family." When it was decided that the number of families served by each community doctor could be doubled, some doctor-nurse teams became responsible for 1,500 or more people. While this degree of primary care coverage was still generous by global standards, the physician-citizen relationship was bound to feel less personal than it had in the past. The number of people covered by each polyclinic was also increased, with between 30,000 and 60,000 included in a polyclinic area as opposed to 20,000 to 40,000 in the past.

Matilde, 56, a senior doctor in Camagüey who had also served on foreign missions, explained to a *Boston Globe* reporter in 2005, "Before, we had a doctor in every factory, every school, every preschool. They were frankly underutilized. We've eliminated a lot of doctors at midlevel administrative desk jobs, and it's probably a leaner, more efficient system now." Her explanation was not likely to satisfy some residents of Havana, who complained to the same reporter that it was getting more difficult to see neighborhood doctors who had once been immediately available.[15] Havana residents I talked with in 2009 said this had definitely been true in some areas, but that problems were gradually being rectified. They credited neighborhood groups and local delegates in the municipal assemblies for being vigilant as they pressed for adequate and balanced medical coverage under the reorganization of doctor-nurse teams. Even with 20,000 doctors working abroad, Cuba had enough remaining at home, about 55,000 in 2009, to serve its entire population more than adequately: there were 4.9 physicians per 1000 citizens, twice as many as in the United States.

Biotech and Bio-Results

Cuban expertise in medicine extends far beyond its abilities to provide primary care and educate community doctors, for it has made a big impact on the world of vaccines and hi-tech drugs and has entered into production agreements with many foreign partners. When the World Health Organization announced that most of Africa was at risk from deadly meningitis outbreaks in 2010, Cuba and Brazil were ready with the capacity to manufacture 50 million doses of the only vaccine in the world that effectively neutralizes the type B meningococcal bacteria. After Cuban scientists had developed the vaccine at the Finlay Institute in Havana, Brazil invested with Cuba in a co-owned, high-volume production plant that became operational in 2007 and soon was capable of meeting large-scale threats in the developing world.

The Cuban Center for Molecular Immunology (CIM) outside of Havana has developed a number of promising anti-cancer drugs, including Nimotuzumab, a monoclonal antibody that has been proven effective in fighting neck, head, and brain tumors and has shown great potential for combating a number of other life-threatening tumors. It was clinically tested, then manufactured for patient applications in joint efforts with companies in India, China, and other countries. Unfortunately it was kept out of clinical tests in the United States by the U.S. embargo until 2009 when a Canadian company, YM Biosciences, was granted a license to begin trials with researchers at U.S. medical centers. Export sales of all Cuban biotech products, which include over 1,200 patents, were worth more than $340 million in 2008, an increase of 20 percent over the previous year. Luis Herrera, head of the Center for Genetic Engineering and Biotechnology (CIGB), believes the fast development of the biotech industry was facilitated by the intense cooperation between all Cuban research institutions: "From the start we realized that we were too poor to indulge in competition with each other."[16] Among many other successes, CIGB produced a vaccine to fight hepatitis B, which had been responsible for a significant amount of liver disease on the island, and within eight years had completely eliminated all early childhood cases of the disease.

These research institutions, which are highly respected in the field of high-tech international drug production, had their beginnings in the 1980s. They managed to survive during the Special Period of the 1990s despite the economic depression and the difficulty of investing in sophisticated laboratory equipment and production facilities. Although money for physical resources was often in short supply, the government had the foresight to keep expanding its human capital by educating more and more highly trained laboratory scientists and then supporting them at the research institutes. Because scientific development was concentrated around one area of west Havana, the country emerged from the economic devastation of the Special Period with highly capable research centers that attracted the attention of companies and nations around the world that were interested in joint ventures. Now the biotech industry has become such an important part of Cuba's international trade that new research centers known as "scientific poles" have been developed in twelve different provinces of the country to facilitate new kinds of cooperation of scientists, professors, and business innovators.

Whereas Cuban scientific research has been impressive, it is the steady attention to every citizen's well-being, especially in the years when the nation could barely feed its people, that has given this relatively poor country the health results of a very rich country. Even with its technological advances, Cuba cannot offer everyone the sophisticated treatments and surgical interventions that are available in the biggest U.S. medical centers. Although it has developed excellent care in orthopedic surgery and many other specialties, Cuba is often unable to afford the newest equipment or medications developed in the rich countries, and the U.S. economic blockade has made it impossible or very difficult to import many essential drugs and supplies. Despite the shortages in Cuba, overall outcomes in terms of mortality compare well with the United States. Although the United States has a tiny edge in years lived for men and women, seventy-nine years in the United States and seventy-eight in Cuba, Cuba has lower rates of mortality for infants and children under five. According to the World Health Organization, the infant mortality rate dropped from eleven to five per thousand in Cuba, while in the United States it decreased from ten to seven. Mortality of children under five years old also dropped by more than half in Cuba, from thirteen to six per thousand, while in the United States, it fell from eleven to eight.[17]

Doctor José Luis Fernández Yero, Director of the Immunoassay Center, Havana, succinctly described why Cuban community-based health care works:

Assessments of the social determinants of health reveal that poor people, uneducated people and people living in marginalized neighborhoods are more likely to get sick and to die than those who are better off. This tells us that everywhere efforts should prioritize these people's health through prevention strategies, supported by appropriate technologies. In our experience, sustainable health depends more on health promotion and disease prevention—including application of technologies for broad health coverage that are appropriate for the socioeconomic environment—than on application of complex technologies or the latest models advertised by market-driven transnational manufacturers. . . . Take infant mortality in Cuba as a health outcome: in 2008, it dropped to below 5 deaths per 1,000 live births. We don't have the same high-tech capabilities as the United States or Canada, but we have lower infant mortality—in part because we have been able to bring the necessary technology closer to all pregnant women and newborns.[18]

5. Barrio Adentro

Some day, therefore, medicine will have to convert itself into a science . . . to provide public health services for the greatest possible number of persons, institute a program of preventive medicine, and orient the public to the performance of hygienic practices. . . . But now old questions reappear: How does one actually carry out a work of social welfare?

—CHE GUEVARA, *On Revolutionary Medicine*, 1960

In 2004, on my first trip to Venezuela, I was picked up at the Caracas airport by a young emergency care doctor, Michel. He was doing a favor for his sister Marcela, a radio reporter who was to be one of my guides around Caracas over the following two weeks. Michel chose to take a detour along the coast, driving past Monte Avila, the long mountain that rises out of the sea to form a 7,000-foot wall between the Caribbean and Caracas. He pointed out the ruins and debris along the deep ravines in the mountainside, the site of tremendous mudslides that buried tens of thousands of people in 1999, the first year of Hugo Chávez's presidency. Many others, almost all of them poor, had been rendered homeless when their shacks were wiped out by the avalanche. Some of those people were still without homes in 2004, and we noticed twenty-five or thirty people gathering inside two broken concrete walls and stoking a small fire with scrap wood and trash. Michel pointed toward the rich apartment towers and luxurious houses that lined the narrow coastal strip, an area about a quarter-mile wide where almost no one had been killed. Almost all the structures were untouched by the mudslides and remained in nice condition; I have since been told by people in the neighborhood that most of these places are still owned by the upper classes, but have seldom been used since 1999. This disaster was the legacy of the old Venezuela, a metaphor for the larger social disaster of a country that had the means to support all of its citizens decently but had degenerated into a place where the rich and upper middle class lived in comfort while the majority were doomed to erect flimsy shacks in perilous places that no one should ever have to inhabit.

"And what happened with health care?" I asked.

"It's even worse," Michel informed me. His emergency room in a public hospital in Caracas never had enough supplies and he and his colleagues were overworked and underpaid. "My hospital is terrible. No, worse than that, abominable. Our public hospitals have been neglected for at least twenty-five years."

Then why did he support Chávez? "Because we need a public health system that works, that cares for everyone." Michel guessed that only about 20 percent of the physicians in Venezuela agreed with him, and that most of those were people like him, working in some capacity within the decrepit old public health system. He hoped that the renovation of hospitals like his own would one day be a well-financed priority, but he had no problem with the fact that the Chávez government had concentrated its efforts on bringing thousands of Cuban doctors to the country over the previous year. "We need them to deliver primary care in the barrios because there are hardly any family doctors for the poor. This is the logical first step in building an equitable, universal system. The doctors at the private clinics that serve the rich and the middle class have no interest in serving the majority of the population."

A Health Care Crisis

Dr. Miguel Requena, dean of the medical school at Central University of Venezuela in Caracas, the nation's premier university, had emphasized the same point in an interview with the *Wall Street Journal* in 2003. He said the Cubans were absolutely necessary to fill the need for general practitioners in rural and urban primary-care clinics because Venezuelan graduates, his own students, were unwilling to do so. "Almost all the new doctors," he said, "want to live in Caracas and other big cities and engage in lucrative specialties, such as plastic surgery."[1]

The old network of elite university medical schools in Venezuela had been producing qualified doctors throughout the 1990s, graduating about 1,200 to 1,500 per year. After graduation, more than half of them went directly into private practice, and another 10 percent were leaving the country in hope of working in more lucrative markets, especially in Spain. Only some 4,000 physicians, about 10 percent of all doctors in the country, were practicing in primary care or family medicine of any kind, and of these just 1,500 were working in deteriorating public clinics.[2]

In the 1960s, Venezuelan governments had aspirations of building a viable public health system based on rudimentary facilities called *ambulatorios* or *consultorios,* small walk-in consulting offices that were located in both urban and rural areas. But as successive governments fell victim to falling oil prices and were party to rising corruption, the economy and society failed to sustain these efforts. One of the obvious reasons for the poor staffing and crumbling structures was diminishing resources: from 1970 to 1996 government funding for health decreased from 13.3 percent of the federal budget to 7.89 percent. A report from the Pan American Health Organization (PAHO) concluded: "Throughout the 1990s, the capability of the public health network to provide health services and resolve health problems became critically insufficient."[3]

By 1998, the year Hugo Chávez was elected, 17 million people out of a population of 24 million had no regular access to medical care.

Adding to the health problems was the shocking shortage of food for the nation's children. Over 4 million children and adolescents suffered from malnutrition, and 1.2 million suffered from severe malnutrition. The situation did not improve fast enough during the early years of Chávez's presidency, so drastic measures were required according to the former Venezuelan Minister of Higher Education, Héctor Navarro. He explained to reporter Claudia Jardim in 2004 that there was a shortage of at least 20,000 physicians and 70 percent of the population lacked regular medical attention. "We have," he said, "a humanitarian crisis on our hands."[4]

Economic and Political Background

The failure of the previous governments to keep contributing to public health care was exacerbated by the fact that half of the population was living in poverty in 1998, and 20.3 percent of them were in extreme poverty. Moses Naim, a fierce critic of Chávez in recent years who resides in the United States and serves as editor of *Foreign Policy* magazine, was Venezuela's Minister of Trade and Industry from 1989 to 1990. Nevertheless, he has acknowledged just how bad economic performance had been before Chávez assumed power; in a 2001 article, he wrote: "In the past 20 years, critical poverty has increased threefold and poverty in general has more than doubled. . . . Real wages are 70 percent below what they were in 1980."[5]

Materially, things did not get much better for the Venezuelan people during Hugo Chávez's first three years in office, 1999–2001. During this time, low prices for oil on the world market and other factors kept the economy in a state of low growth and stagnation. Furthermore, Chávez has not been able to consolidate a political majority among the national legislature or the nations' governors and was constantly opposed by a Supreme Court that followed the wishes of big business. One bright spot was that a   broad spectrum of the Venezuelan people participated in a constitutional convention in 1999 and approved one of the most progressive democratic constitutions in the world. According to Venezuelan political analyst Eva Golinger, this was "the first and foremost important achievement during the Chávez administration. . . . The 1999 Constitution was, in fact, drafted—written—by the people of Venezuela in one of the most participatory examples of nation building, and then was ratified through popular national referendum by 75 percent of Venezuelans. The 1999 Constitution is one of the most advanced in the world in the area of human rights. It guarantees the rights to housing, education, health care, food, indigenous lands, languages, women's rights, worker's rights, living wages, and a whole host of other rights that few other countries recognize on a national level. My favorite right in the Venezuelan Constitution is the right to a dignified life."[6]

The rights to health care are spelled out in specific articles of the Bolivarian Constitution, Articles 82 through 86, which define access to medical care as a fundamental right of all citizens. The articles give the government the responsibility of providing and financing a universal and participatory public health system.

In 2001, President Chávez utilized this new constitution to enact a series of laws and programs that sowed panic in the hearts of the Venezuelan oligarchy. Among these were provisions that would allow the government to create *misiones sociales*, or social missions, including the Barrio Adentro medical program, that would greatly improve the lives of poor and working-class people in the years to come. But as far as the rich were concerned there were much more worrisome measures that affected them immediately in 2001. They feared legal limits to their unbridled pursuit of property and wealth under new laws that concerned land reform and the distribution of oil industry revenues. Other laws changed the tax structure or simply directed the government to take sterner measures in collecting taxes that had been going unpaid for years. The oligarchy and business establishment decided to act quickly before these changes could be implemented.

From late 2001 to early 2003, the oligarchy made repeated attempts to dislodge Chávez and his administration. A spate of economic disruptions preceded a coup d'état in April 2002 that was concocted by big business and some military generals, with the encouragement of pressure groups financed by the United States. The coup removed Chávez from power, but only for a little more than twenty-four hours. It failed because the majority of the military and millions of the poor rallied to President Chávez's defense. In the months immediately after the attempted coup, almost no coup participants were arrested as Chávez made a number of conciliatory gestures toward the business community and his political opponents. These were interpreted as signs of weakness by the oligarchy, and three attempts at economic sabotage were then launched by the big business confederation, Fedecameras. It tried to cripple the country by closing businesses and factories, in hope that the desperate state of the economy would make it impossible for Chávez to govern. Fedecameras's machinations culminated in the devastating management strike that shut down the state-owned oil business, Petroleos de Venezuela, S.A., usually known as PDVSA, in December of 2002 and January of 2003. The acts of sabotage instigated by senior executives and corrupt union bosses led to the halt of almost all oil exports. Although Chávez was able to withstand these attacks, the shocks to the Venezuelan economy were catastrophic. Gross domestic product fell about 16 percent in 2002 and 2003 and contributed to an even further increase in national poverty levels. Nearly two-thirds of the population, or 62.1 percent, were living in poverty, and almost one-third, 29.8 percent, were living in extreme poverty.

Economic and Social Change Under Chávez, 2003–2008

Chávez reacted to the sabotage of the oil industry by throwing out the top management of PDVSA and thousands of senior employees who had cooperated with the shutdown. The new directors appointed by Chávez consolidated control over the oil revenues and began investing the profits directly in social projects that benefited the Venezuelan people. This investment helped the Venezuelan economy achieve remarkable growth over the next six years, from mid-2003 through

2008, and allowed the Chávez government to completely reverse the
direction of the country. The poverty rate, 62.1 percent in 2003, was
cut in half, to 31.5 percent in 2008. The extreme poverty rate
declined by two-thirds, from 29.5 percent to 9.5 percent.[7] The Gross
domestic product grew by 78 percent, and average income grew by
more than 50 percent in real terms, that is, after adjusting for high
rates of inflation. (This figure has been confirmed by the CIA's
"country report" for Venezuela, which cites per capita incomes of
$8,000 in 1998 and $13,500 in 2008.)

In addition to strong economic growth during this period, there
was a remarkable redistribution of income, due mainly to growing
employment opportunities and generous increases in the minimum
wage mandated by the government. Though most upper-income
groups did not suffer income losses, the lower 80 to 90 percent of the
population made much larger income gains. The private company
Datanalysis, which generally issues statistical studies for the country's
business associations, reported income gains of 445 percent for the
Venezuelan lower classes, versus 194 percent for the upper classes
from 1998 to 2006.[8] These income gains for the majority meant that
the Gini coefficient, a standard economic measure of the degree of
economic inequality, declined dramatically from .39 to .49 between
1999 and 2010. This was a substantial reduction, especially in so
short a time. One way to illustrate the impact of this change is by
looking at a similar large movement in the Gini index of inequality, but
in the opposite direction, from 40.3 to 46.9, that occurred in the
United States.[9] This shift, which took place over a longer time, from
1980 to 2005, transferred a huge amount of income to the top 1 percent of the U.S. population, who saw their share of national income
jump from 9 percent to 22 percent, while the income share of the huge
majority of working people, the bottom 90 percent of the population,
declined precipitously from 65 percent to 50 percent.

In addition to the growth in real incomes for the whole population,
which are only generally calculated in cash figures according to
salaries earned, there were also other significant economic gains for
the majority of Venezuelans. These gains cannot be calculated in exact

monetary terms, but they certainly have raised the standard of living of
the 80 percent of the population who would be considered poor and
working class. These new social "wages" contribute greatly to the
egalitarian direction that Venezuelan society has taken under Chávez
because they go disproportionately to the poorer citizens. Social
spending makes up a staggering share of the gross domestic product.
According to economists Mark Weisbrot and Luis Sandoval, "The
central government's social spending has increased massively, from
8.2 percent of the gross domestic product in 1998 to 13.6 percent for
2006; in real (inflation-adjusted) terms, social spending per person
has increased by 170 percent over the period 1998-2006." They
report that this is not the true extent of social spending in Venezuela,
because many expenditures are not recorded in the central government figures. Billions of dollars for the social missions flow directly
from the coffers of the national oil industry, PDVSA; this contribution
by itself amounted to 7.3 percent of GDP in 2006. With this included,
"social spending reached 20.9 percent of GDP in 2006, at least 314
percent more than in 1998 (in terms of real, inflation-adjusted social
spending per person)."[10]

Among the many non-cash sources of income supplied through the
social missions and not accounted for in assessing income redistribution are free health care, free education programs, free food for millions
of children at school and the most impoverished adults, heavily subsidized food available at more than 15,000 Mercal food stores, tens of
thousands of free neighborhood recreation and sports programs, free
housing grants or interest-free loans, and free work-training programs.
In addition there are a great many public works that often benefit poor
and working-class people more than the rich, such as the new subway
and bus lines added to the Caracas public transportation system.

Barrio Adentro Begins

After the economic and political assaults in 2002-03 had nearly
wrecked the economy, it took a few years for the Chávez administra-

tion to achieve the large income gains cited above. In contrast, the Venezuelan government was able to immediately embark upon many of the social missions mandated in the new constitution. Although the political determination of President Chávez was important in implementing decisive improvements in education, health care, and other social areas, two other factors were decisive: the Venezuelan government's direct control of oil revenues and its close relationship with Cuba. On October 30, 2000, the original Cuba-Venezuela Comprehensive Cooperation Agreement was signed by Fidel Castro and Hugo Chávez. It allowed for a growing exchange of goods, services, and expertise between the two countries, with Venezuela's largest contribution being petroleum, starting with 53,000 barrels per day in 2001 and growing to almost 100,000 barrels per day by 2007, a level maintained through 2010. Cuba reciprocated with its major resource, human capital: thousands of teachers, agronomists, technicians, and other experts, who aided in reconstructing Venezuelan society. By 2009, this bilateral exchange, which had hardly existed during the 1990s ($30 million per year in trade), was valued at over $3 billion according to Venezuelan Minister of Economy Ali Rodriguez.

Once the Chávez government consolidated control of the revenues of the state oil company PDVSA in early 2003, it could sustain the large investment in the social missions that became the heart and soul of the Bolivarian Revolution. The flagship program of all the social missions was Barrio Adentro, made possible by the Convenio de Cooperacion Integral de Salud, the Agreement of Comprehensive Cooperation in Health. This allowed for the largest and most important contingent of Cuban volunteers, health professionals, to come to Venezuela.

In 2002, in the midst of all the political strife, the Venezuelan government was making plans to deliver free public health care to every neighborhood in the country that did not have adequate medical facilities. According to Luis Montiel Araujo, a physician with Venezuela's Ministry of Health and Social Development, "Barrio Adentro was conceived as a way to bring medical services to the excluded . . . to put a physician in every community." The words *barrio adentro,* meaning "inside the neighborhood," were taken literally; that is, public health doctors really were expected to go *inside* the barrios, not only to attend to residents but to live among the people. (The word *barrio* has a distinct meaning in Venezuela, where it connotes a large district made up of smaller neighborhoods of poor and working-class people. Wealthy and upper-middle-class neighborhoods are not barrios.) In this planning phase, the government issued a call for Venezuelan physicians to volunteer. "They were not receptive," said Dr. Montiel. About 50 doctors answered this call and when the program actually got under way the following year, only 29 Venezuelan doctors were participating.[11]

At the time, Freddy Bernal was the mayor of Libertador, a large municipality in the city of Caracas with a population of 1.5 million people, most of them poor and working class. With the support of the Ministry of Health, Bernal decided to circumvent the shortage of Venezuelan doctors and make the pilot program of Barrio Adentro operational by employing outside help. In April of 2003, at Bernal's invitation, fifty-four Cuban doctors arrived to open the offices of Barrio Adentro in Libertador. In May, another hundred Cuban doctors came, and by July there were 627 working in the municipality's barrios. At this point, the national government decided Barrio Adentro was a project worthy of immediate replication in six other states of Venezuela: Zulia, Lara, Trujillo, Vargas, Miranda, and Barinas. By October, a total of 2,000 Cuban physicians had taken up residence throughout Venezuela, some even settling in remote rural areas.

About this time, a Venezuelan physician who was in charge of an older public clinic in Caracas, Dr. Rosa Martinson, explained to reporters Argiris Malapanis and Camilo Catalán why the Cubans were necessary. Her clinic could serve only one-third of the patients it was capable of handling because the other Venezuelan doctors who had been assigned to work with her seldom showed up. "For them, it's offensive to work in the barrio. They'd rather work in the Caracas central hospital. They say this neighborhood is ugly. They look at the people here as dirty, smelly, and dangerous."[12]

The Cuban doctors who reported for work in Venezuela saw poor people in a different light. The desperate circumstances of many Venezuelans were the object of their humanitarian concern rather than something to be avoided. One of the new arrivals, Nilda Collazo, began working in a remote part of the western state of Lara in July of 2003. Later that year she told visiting reporters, "Up here you find diseases long eradicated in our country. It's rare to find a child who doesn't suffer from parasites or a pregnant woman who has even once seen a doctor. . . . It's a picture that brings out your human sensibilities." Collazo gained instant hero status in her area when a child was bitten by a poisonous snake in the isolated hamlet of Los Portones. Since no vehicle was available, Dr. Collazo wrapped the girl in a blanket, walked three hours to the nearest hospital, and the child survived.[13]

In Los Potocos, 150 miles to the other side of Caracas in the east, doctors were seeing the same effects of social neglect. "This is the first time I've left Cuba, and I'd never seen anything like this," said Leonardo Hernandez, a twenty-seven-year-old doctor. When he and his colleagues arrived in 2003, they found malnourished children and widespread diarrhea. By 2005, he told an Associated Press reporter, children were demonstrably healthier due to rudimentary care, more food and vitamins, and much better sanitation.[14]

Any visitor to Venezuela who has also visited other Latin American countries cannot help but notice that upper-middle-class Venezuelans, perhaps as much as 10 percent of the population, do not seem to live in a developing country. For decades they have lived as comfortably as people in the advanced capitalist countries, and they identify strongly with the consumer culture of the United States. One of their favorite activities in the past was flying to Miami on shopping trips.

The working and lower classes, however, do not resemble those in the United States or any other developed nation. A large swath of the lower classes has suffered indignities and afflictions common to those suffered by their counterparts in the poorest parts of Africa and Latin America. Thus, when the more experienced Cuban physicians arrived in Venezuela in 2003, they found the same ailments they had seen on their missions to the poorest countries of the world, nations whose per capita GDP was but a fraction of the $8,000 average in Venezuela at the time. For example, in the Americas, Cuban doctors were attending to poor people in nations such as Honduras and Haiti ($2,050 and $1,340 GDP per capita, respectively), and in Africa even poorer places, Ethiopia ($560) and Angola ($1,030).[15]

The Evolving Structure of Barrio Adentro

Barrio Adentro expanded at an astounding rate in its first year and a half of existence, growing from a trial program in Caracas in the spring of 2003 to a nationwide network of 13,000 physicians working in all twenty-four states of Venezuela by the fall of 2004. It was reported that there were 8,500 primary care *consultorios populares,* popular consultation offices, in operation. This was a rough approximation because the first facilities were often in temporary quarters, carved out of any available space in the neighborhoods. Vacant storefronts and empty rooms in families' homes were utilized; corners of churches, schools, and public buildings were freed up for temporary use; and empty *ambulatorios* from the old public system were once again employed as walk-in primary care clinics.[16]

The process of accommodating the medical personnel from Cuba required an immense amount of effort from Venezuelans, and gave many formerly marginalized residents of the barrios their first experience of being active participants in the Bolivarian Revolution. As the doctors and other health workers began work, the first neighborhood health committees were forming in barrios and villages. Each neighborhood of 1,500 to 2,000 people that wanted a Cuban doctor to serve them was expected to organize a committee of ten to twenty volunteers from the community who would commit themselves to finding office spaces, providing sleeping quarters, collecting furniture and simple fixtures, and feeding the medical providers. The health committees were also there to support the doctors in other ways, such as accompanying them on house-to-house visits, helping them compile data on health problems, malnutrition, and chronic diseases, and joining in public health campaigns to educate their neighbors about preventive care and healthy living.

Barrio Adentro doctors saw patients every morning at their consulting offices and traversed the neighborhoods every afternoon, meeting people, inquiring about family health, and treating those who were reluctant to visit the clinics. Generally, the Cuban physicians lived in spartan rooms attached to the Barrio Adentro offices or in the homes of nearby residents, so that they would be available for emergency visits twenty-four hours a day, seven days a week. This kind of medical attention was something the people they served had never experienced. Prior to 2003, there were just 1,500 doctors employed by the Venezuelan government to provide primary care in a public system that had 4,400 offices called *ambulatorios*. The small number of attending physicians meant that many of these walk-in offices were virtually empty, often staffed only one or two days a week by doctors, or only by nurses.

In the six years after Barrio Adentro was founded, the number of *consultorios* decreased by about 20 percent, since some temporary facilities that were no longer necessary were closed down and the system was consolidated and organized throughout 335 municipalities in all twenty-four states of Venezuela.[17] In October of 2009, President Chávez used his Sunday television show, *"Alo Presidente,"* to sum up the achievements of Barrio Adentro over the previous six years. He reported that the government had 6,711 *consultorios populares* serving patients in city neighborhoods and rural villages.[18] These form Barrio Adentro I, the first stage of comprehensive community care, which offers free primary care to any citizen who seeks it. Nearly half of the consulting offices, 3,249 of them, were located in newly constructed buildings called *modulos*. These modules are the distinctive small, octagonal, two-story red brick structures that can be seen in most barrios in the large cities and some rural settings.

According to the president, the *consultorios populares* were staffed by 6,323 Cuban specialists in comprehensive general medicine in 2009 and 1,641 Venezuelan doctors who had completed their two-year residencies in this specialty while working in Barrio Adentro I. The number of primary care doctors, slightly under 8,000, was significantly lower than the 13,000 who had staffed the provisional Barrio

Adentro offices in 2004, but this was because the Barrio Adentro system had been gradually evolving into different tiers of organized care. By October of 2009, there were 5,296 Cuban physicians working in other capacities, most of them specialists working at the diagnostic centers of Barrio Adentro II, and the rest in educational, supervisory, and other specialist roles.

Another important feature of Barrio Adentro I was the provision of dental care. Though not as numerous as the ambulatory medical clinics, Barrio Adentro dental offices also had a profound impact on the health of poor communities. As was the case with primary medical care, there had been attempts by past Venezuelan governments to provide some dental care at public facilities; in 2002 there were 2,371 Venezuelan dentists employed by the Social Security Service and the Ministry of Health, but their level of productivity, in terms of patients treated, was very low. As was the case with primary medical care before Chávez became president, diminishing government expenditures on health care caused the provision of public dental care to deteriorate. A great many dentists employed by the government devoted only a limited number of hours to their public service jobs because they were trying to expand their opportunities in the more lucrative area of private practice.

At the end of 2003, three Cuban dentists started a trial program in a Caracas barrio and, in little more than a year, were joined by 3,000 of their compatriots who were dispersed to every state of Venezuela. By 2009, there were over 1,600 Barrio Adentro dentistry offices operating with 4,767 dentists at work, including 2,683 Cubans and 2,084 Venezuelans. Among the Venezuelans, some had worked in the old public programs and others were recent graduates of traditional Venezuelan dental schools who completed their residencies in comprehensive general dentistry by working alongside experienced Cuban dentists. Although the new staffing level was only twice as high as in the old government dentistry programs, the Barrio Adentro dentistry offices were treating ten times as many patients as the old system.

Since medical care is not delivered by doctors and dentists alone, there were also many other Cubans working at the various levels of

Barrio Adentro. Figures provided by the Cuban Medical Mission for 2008 show that there were 4,158 nurses in Venezuela, most with a university level of education. Approximately 7,500 highly trained medical technicians were working in laboratories, imaging, rehabilitation, and other specialties. Optical technicians operated 459 optometry offices, where any Venezuelan could go to be fitted for free eyeglasses. Finally, there were over 5,000 sports trainers working in cooperation with the medical personnel in neighborhood centers, schools, and other Bolivarian facilities.

Secondary Treatment and Barrio Adentro II

From the beginning of the Venezuelan-Cuban cooperative health agreement, it was clear that Barrio Adentro II was essential to the functioning of Barrio Adentro I, since primary treatment networks must be joined to a more sophisticated grid of secondary clinics. Beginning in 2004, the Chávez government started effectively locating and constructing a secondary system of Barrio Adentro II diagnostic clinics or CDIs (Clinicas Diagnosticas Integrales), each of which is designed to serve a group of ten to twenty of the neighborhood walk-in consultation offices with sophisticated treatment and analysis that cannot be provided at the neighborhood level. These are sizable facilities with emergency units, offices for specialists, rooms for a variety of modern laboratory and imaging equipment, and a limited number of hospital beds, usually six to twelve, for intensive care patients and seriously ill people who cannot be transferred to a larger hospital. The government's goal in 2004 was to incorporate 600 CDIs into the Bolivarian health system; in October of 2009, they were staffed by more than 4,477 Cuban physicians, several hundred Venezuelan doctors, and thousands of technicians and nurses from both countries. By 2011, there were 533 CDIs in operation.

The plans for Barrio Adentro II in 2004 provided for two other important components: 35 Centers of High Technology and 600 Comprehensive Rehabilitation Rooms. The high technology centers, known as Centros de Alta Technologia, or CAT, provide complex clinical laboratory tests and diagnostic support services such as nuclear magnetic resonance, computerized axial tomography, 3-D ultrasound, mammography, video endoscopy, and electro-cardiography. The rehabilitation rooms, known as Salones de Rehabilitacion Integral, or SRI, provide physical therapy of various kinds. The SRIs are spacious facilities built to accompany each diagnostic clinic and located in separate wings or in nearby buildings. They offer sophisticated regimens using exercise machines, hydrotherapy, electrotherapy, and acupuncture, under the guidance of experienced Cuban rehabilitation technicians, with Venezuelans in training alongside them. Most of these also offer a variety of alternative therapies such as acupuncture and electronic stimulation. By early 2011, 31 CAT facilities and 570 SRI rooms were completed and functioning.[19]

On a brief visit to Venezuela in January of 2009, I talked with Gaudy Garcia, a schoolteacher in her late fifties. She had earned her university degree after thirty years of working as a campesina in the steep fields outside the village of Monte Carmelo. Because she had been suffering bouts of severe leg and back pain, her Barrio Adentro doctor prescribed a series of twenty-one rehabilitation treatments—for one hour, three times a week—at the rehab center that is attached to the back of the diagnostic clinic in the nearby town of Sanare. Gaudy said, laughing, "It's like I get three vacations per week. I love the water treatment and the nurses and rehab specialists are fun, we joke all the time. But they're serious, too, they make sure I am doing all the proper exercises to recover my strength."

A More Challenging Step, Barrio Adentro III

The most difficult task in creating the new public health system in Venezuela has been the development of Barrio Adentro III, which involves improving the nation's existing public hospital system. These facilities had been neglected and deteriorating for at least twenty years before Hugo Chávez took power, but were forced to wait for attention while the basic levels of Barrio Adentro were being formed. It was not until June of 2005, more than two years after Barrio Adentro I began, that the Venezuelan government announced the formation of Barrio Adentro III: "This mission has an integral goal that includes: modernizing and updating medical technology, changing the model of assistance, restructuring the management model from which synergy can be promoted, promoting community participation and constructing new hospitals to guarantee access to medical attention for all citizens." In 2006, forty-two hospitals serving 60 percent of the population were chosen for upgrades, and by 2008 this program was extended to more than ninety hospitals, with the final goal being to fix all 300 public hospitals in the country.

The delay in starting reconstruction of the hospital system was due to a conscious choice by the medical experts who designed Barrio Adentro; they wanted to concentrate on building a public, free, and universal health system from the ground up, that is, starting with primary care delivery at the neighborhood level. This was achieved quickly, although in an ad hoc manner, because 14,000 Cuban doctors were prepared to work and live in rather primitive conditions, and because neighborhood volunteers put so much effort into providing them with shelter, food, and makeshift quarters for medical practice.

Fixing the old hospitals, equipping them with new technology, building new ones, and coordinating the work with other parts of the health networks was by necessity a much more lengthy and expensive undertaking. Not only did it require extraordinary planning and allocation of resources, but it was complicated by a tangled web of conflicting obligations in the old system. Bureaucratic structures of the past—such as the Governors' Offices, the IVSS (Venezuelan Social Security Institute), PDVSA (Petroleos de Venezuela), the Military Health System, IPASME (Institute for Prevention and Social Assistance for the Employees of the Ministry of Education), the federal government's Ministry of Health—still existed, and they all had their own hospital networks and distinct systems of hiring and compensating medical professionals. Reconstruction and reorganization required special arrangements to keep things functioning; for instance, military hospitals, judged by many to be those that maintained the best quality of care during previous decades, were asked to treat many civilian patients who had no connection to the military services.

The inefficiencies of the old hospital bureaucracies were exacerbated by lack of public oversight at the state and local levels, as many renovation and new construction projects went over budget, fell behind schedule, and were left uncompleted. On top of this, Venezuela was hit hard by the worldwide economic recession of 2008-09 that caused petroleum prices to fall dramatically along with the revenues that the government could devote to this multi-billion-dollar project. Some hospitals, often the most needy ones, suffered from shortages of supplies and medications, as well as the breakdown of medical equipment, and had difficulty delivering proper care to their patients. With the world economy emerging from recession in 2010 and petroleum prices rising, the Chávez government was able to push through more projects to completion and begin to confront one of the biggest underlying problems.

In February 2011, the Minister of Health, Dr. Eugenia Sader, reported to the National Assembly that 148 of the major hospital projects had been completed since 1998, and that her ministry had been pushing more diligently for completion of other projects. She emphasized that many of these projects were still incomplete because of the dishonest dealings of private companies. Building contractors had received full payment in advance and left the work half finished, she said, and the government was now going to issue warrants for their arrest. This uncompromising response by Dr. Sader and the Chávez government was unusual and very promising. It was a sign that they were ready to fight the worst enemy of the revolutionary process, the graft and corruption that have been endemic to Venezuelan society for so long that it seemed that no government, including the Bolivarian one, could weed them out.[20]

Barrio Adentro IV

The fourth component of the new system is the construction of fifteen highly specialized hospitals that focus on research and the most advanced forms of treatment for specific medical problems and patients. One of the first to be completed in August 2007 was the Dr. Gilberto Rodríguez Ochoa Latin American Children's Cardiology Hospital in Caracas, a state-of-the-art facility that has aspirations of being the finest of its kind in Latin America. Other hospitals, including those specializing in oncology, nephrology, gastroenterology, and adult cardiology, were slated for construction in the states of Guarico, Apure, Merida, Miranda, and Barinas. These projects were delayed by budget constraints due to the recession of 2008–09, but regained momentum in 2010. Although Barrio IV appears to be less prone to corruption than Barrio III, its construction efforts have been criticized by both the political opposition, who don't like this kind of high-end expenditure on public medicine, and some Chávez supporters, who contend that the first order of business is spending these funds to complete the more low-tech, preventive side of a universal medical system.

Barrio Adentro's Accomplishments

Within the overall context of economic growth, income redistribution, and social spending, BolivarianVenezuela has been able to radically reverse the falling government investment in health care. Venezuelan health spending as a percentage of the GDP increased from 2.8 percent in 1997 to 6 percent in 2007.[21] This figure was heading higher when the world economic recession caused the Venezuelan economy to stagnate at the end of 2008 and limited the expansion of social missions. By 2009, the number of people utilizing the new health care system revolving around Barrio Adentro was impressive. Research polls showed that 82 percent of the population were using the services of public medical personnel and facilities. More than 75 percent were satisfied with the service according to INE, the National Statistics Institute. The large majority of people who were paying for private health insurance and private clinics reported that they were also happy with their service, too, but they constituted only 18 percent of the population.[22]

The government's determination to make the public health system accessible to all has led to tremendous increases in the number of patients served. From the 1998 figure of 3.5 million patient visits, public health service began to grow rapidly, particularly after the introduction of Barrio Adentro in 2003. Between 2004 and 2010 the number of patients seen by doctors in Barrio Adentro I averaged over 60 million per year. Consultations in Barrio Adentro II rose to 15 million per year as more Diagnostic Centers were completed. In October of 2010, President Chávez announced that 482 million consultations had been performed by doctors in Barrio Adentro I and II between April 2003 and the end of August 2010, and that 83 percent of Venezuelans had been served by Barrio Adentro.

The increased medical attention paid off quickly in human terms during the first ten years of the revolution, as infant mortality fell from 19 to 13.9 deaths per 1000 live births between 1999 and 2008 and the mortality of all children under five fell from 26.5 to 16.7. Postneonatal mortality was cut by more than half, falling from 9.0 to 4.2 deaths per 1000 live births. The life span of the average Venezuelan increased by 1.5 years between 2000 and 2009.[23]

Charles Briggs and Clara Mantini-Briggs, anthropologists at the University of California, wrote about Barrio Adentro in 2009, and emphasized that the development of more positive and egalitarian physician-patient and professional-community relationships "may be one of the easiest, most effective ways" the medical profession can contribute to overcoming health disparities." They wrote that the

. . . Misión Barrio Adentro emerged from creative interactions between policymakers, clinicians, community workers, and residents, adopting flexible, problem-solving strategies. In addition, data indi-

cated that egalitarian physician–patient relationships and the direct
involvement of local health committees overcame distrust and generated popular support for the program. Media and opposition antagonism complicated physicians' lives and clinical practices, but height-
ened the program's visibility. Top-down and bottom-up efforts are
less effective than "horizontal" collaborations between professionals
and residents in underserved communities. Direct, local involvement
can generate creative and dynamic efforts to address acute health disparities in these areas.[24]

In short, this academic appraisal emphasized the effectiveness of
Barrio Adentro in delivering primary medical attention and preventive
care to a large, previously unserved population, and gave special
importance to the egalitarian relationships and interactions that build
trust among the common people. When these factors are considered
along with the positive change in health statistics, we have a reasonable
prescription for bringing health care to all.

6. Witnessing Barrio Adentro in Action

His awareness grows that what poor people need is not so much his
scientific knowledge as a doctor, but rather his strength and persist-
ence in trying to bring about the social change that would enable them
to recover the dignity that had been taken from them and trampled on
for centuries. With his thirst for knowledge and his great capacity to
love, he shows us how reality, if properly interpreted, can permeate a
human being to the point of changing his or her way of thinking.

—ALEIDA GUEVARA, Cuban pediatrician,
writing about her father Che

Just a few days after my arrival in Venezuela in November 2004, my
guide Marcela and I met with Juan Ramon Echeverria, a social worker
and lifelong barrio resident, who gave us a short and effective political
and social history of the Caracas barrio of Antímano, emphasizing that
many years of social struggles and protests had developed a progressive political consciousness among the population long before the
Bolivarian Revolution. He led us to one of the *consultorios populares*,
or neighborhood consulting offices, that were scattered all over the
large barrio, a community of 250,000 that lies in the hills on the south
side of the city. This particular *consultorio* was one of a few newly
constructed *modulos*, a two-story octagon built of red tile bricks and

roofed and trimmed with bright blue metal. The distinctive building, easy to spot as a health care outpost, was simple and compact: a waiting room and two consulting/examination rooms on the ground floor and a tiny two-bedroom apartment for a pair of family care doctors on the second floor. The doctors not only worked inside the barrio, they lived inside it as well.

Only about 280 of these new octagonal structures existed in Venezuela at the time, because the government had just begun constructing them that year (by 2010, over 3,200 of the new *modulos* had been erected). But the lack of new facilities had not stopped Barrio Adentro from expanding into almost every municipality in all twenty-four states of Venezuela. Many of the Barrio Adentro locations were temporary: rooms in private homes, vacant storefronts, empty spaces in community buildings and churches. Some of the old *consultorios*, also known as *ambulatorios* or ambulatory clinics, had been created by former governments forty years earlier and then abandoned; now they were occupied again by the Cuban medical staff. At this time, there was activity that would lead to the implementation of the next level of care, Barrio Adentro II, but it was mostly talk. Barrio Adentro II was going to require more sophisticated and larger diagnostic clinics known as Clinicas Diagnosticas Integrales, or CDIs, and Salones de Rehabilitacion, rehabilitation rooms for physical therapy services. As of November 2004, only six of the new CDIs had been built in the country, out of 600 that would eventually be needed.[1]

When we entered the Barrio Adentro modulo, the Cuban doctors were so busy with a long line of patients they did not have time to talk with us. A member of the local health committee said they typically served one hundred people a day, including a few who came from outside the neighborhood and also received care at no charge. She showed us a computer printout taped to one of the walls of the reception area that recorded pertinent statistics about health: 1,712 residents, 82 children suffering from asthma, 92 adults with hypertension. The concern with community well-being was broad, as evidenced by a posting that listed the numbers of employed and unemployed adults in the neighborhood.

From the new octagonal module, we walked farther up the steep hill to another small neighborhood, and here the Barrio Adentro consulting office was simply two bare concrete rooms in the semi-basement of a family's house. The Cuban doctor was taking a vacation back home; she had worked eighteen months without a break. A couple of tables and a tall cabinet were completely bare because everything of value, all medicines and some modest equipment, had been locked up so it wouldn't be stolen when she was away. The doctor's own personal quarters consisted of a tiny bathroom and a bare concrete room furnished only with a small bed, a nightstand, a stool, and a lamp. Juan Ramon Echeverria explained that this setup was typical of many temporary quarters for Barrio Adentro throughout Antímano.

A member of the local health committee told us that their first task had been searching for vacant space, finding the funds to rent it, and furnishing it with donated items. Then she laughed and said, "The second thing we did, when our doctor arrived, was to organize a security detail. This is a rough barrio and not a safe place for a young woman who doesn't know her way around. So we walked everywhere with her, sometimes as many as ten of us at once just to show how much community support there was. It was important to accompany her on house calls, too, because some people were shy or frightened. We were especially concerned that pregnant women were not taking advantage of free checkups because they had heard anti-Cuban propaganda on TV from the political opposition and the Venezuelan medical association. Now they all come regularly and have confidence in her, and she will send them to a diagnostic clinic if there are problems with the pregnancy."

On the way out of the office, we noted once again that there were statistical charts on the wall, this time handwritten by members of the health committee. This is a key reason for the success of Barrio Adentro and the concept of comprehensive community medicine; it demonstrates that neighborhood people were participating in creating a culture of "wellness" from the very beginning. The data on the entire neighborhood, which consisted of 210 families and 1,460 individuals, indicated three ailments that were major problems for the community: children with asthma, adults with hypertension, and both children and adults at risk for diabetes.

In addition to these chronic ailments, there was one immediately preventable condition: malnutrition. There were 150 people in that category, more than 10 percent of the population. In many cases, health committee members had sought these people out in their homes and convinced them to see the doctor when she came on a house call, and then assisted them with treatment. The prescribed treatment, after the doctor had examined them and determined that they were indeed malnourished and did not have the resources for an adequate diet, was to sign them up for two meals per day served by the *casa de alimentación*—literally the "house of nourishment"— a community kitchen that was operated by five neighborhood women out of a private home.

That was our next stop. The government provided the house with extra gas burners, an assortment of large pots, and regular deliveries of quality ingredients from which they prepared an assortment of dishes. The women worked as volunteers, but were entitled to take as much food as they needed for their own families. The food recipients or their caretakers came to the house with their personal array of plastic Tupperware-like dishes and took their meals home. The community kitchen house had only a small sitting room with one dining table, one couch, and a couple of side chairs. I ate the midday meal that had been prepared for everyone else: chicken in a savory sauce, rice, cabbage and carrot salad, *platanos*, and a very rich peach juice. As we said goodbye, the food delivery truck was arriving on the street and neighborhood children were there to greet it. Kids between five and ten years old grabbed bags of garlic, onions, and other vegetables, and started negotiating the narrow, zigzag staircase that passed several houses before descending to the cooks in their kitchen. One of the bigger kids was proud to show that he could lift a huge sack of potatoes that weighed nearly as much as he did and then, with it balanced on his shoulder, hop skillfully down the steps to the kitchen.

The spirit of community involvement, which had been kindled by the success of Barrio Adentro committees, was contagious. It was enabling the neighborhood to organize other efforts that improved the quality of life, such as the public sanitation project that had been undertaken just a couple of months before my visit. Using materials donated by the government, but relying on volunteer labor from the community, residents had dug up the main street and installed a new network of sewer and water pipes. When the work was completed, the municipality repaved the street and left the extra pipes and fittings for the neighborhood's use. These were divided up among the community members who were able to make use of them for their own construction projects, such as bathrooms that still needed to be hooked up to the public sewage system.

Juan Ramon Echeverria explained that this kind of activity never would have been possible in the past, for there had never been neighborhood organizations like the health committee that served everyone. There had been Bolivarian Circles, groups of politicized volunteers who were valuable assets for Chávez's early political campaigns, but they had never developed into a cohesive force that could bring everyone together to define and meet community goals.

As we left the *casa de alimentación,* an old fellow poked his head out of a nearby house. He had once suffered from severe glaucoma and had just come back from having a successful eye operation in Cuba. He was one of the first of more than 200,000 Venezuelans who were flown to Cuba on planes for restorative surgery under a program called Misión Milagro, or Miracle Mission. Later, another 300,000 Venezuelans had various ophthalmologic surgeries performed at new eye clinics established in their own country; by the end of the decade physicians from both Cuba and Venezuela would be performing similar surgery on patients from all over Latin America and the Caribbean.

Next we met a mother, with her eight-year-old son at her side, who explained that he had been wasting away from intense fever, neck aches, and weakness until their Barrio Adentro doctor suspected bacterial meningitis and ordered him to get blood tests at the diagnostic

clinic. The doctor's suspicion was correct, and the boy was hospital-
ized, treated with the proper antibiotics, and fully recovered. "If not,"
said his mother, "I'm sure he would have died."

Dr. Yonel's Army of Peace

That afternoon I finally met my first Cuban medical professional, Dr.
Yonel, a young dentist who had been working in Antímano for about
five months. He said that most Cuban medical personnel were willing
to volunteer for a two-year tour of duty just as he had done, but he
knew some who had family responsibilities and other obligations that
kept them at home and others who simply had no inclination to travel.
"I'm young and single and want to see the world," he said, then added,
"Frankly, the most important reason I'm here is that I dreamed of
being a doctor when I was a little kid, and the real heroes for me were
the Cuban doctors who traveled to other lands to help people, especially to Africa in those days. Before coming here I worked in a polyclinic in Havana with a team of nineteen dentists and they all encouraged me to take advantage of this opportunity."

Someone decided to tease Dr. Yonel, probably because he was
handsome and single. "Don't you like our Venezuelan girls? Maybe
you'll decide to marry one and then where will you live, here or in
Cuba?"

"Well, the girls are very pretty here, and pretty aggressive, too." He
grinned. "I guess I could do either, but my job and my colleagues are
waiting for me in Havana, so I expect that I will return. I'm not sure a
Venezuelan woman would be prepared to live there, since the wife of
a Cuban doctor cannot expect to have many material possessions."

Earlier, a woman in the health committee at the first Barrio
Adentro I had visited, the spiffy octagonal module, had explained that
when the first doctors arrived in Antímano, the neighborhood health
committee feared for their safety and insisted that members accompany the physicians wherever they went and act as bodyguards. When
asked about this, Dr. Yonel said, "There is a level of street crime here

that is hard for us Cubans to comprehend, so of course I take precautions that I would not worry about in Havana. At first, our barrio neighbors had fears that opposition political forces would harass us, but I have never had any problems." He came to the barrio a year after the first Cuban arrivals, and felt comfortable exploring the city on his own, visiting various museums and the Central University, and talking freely with many Venezuelans, even a few who were opposed to President Chávez.

Still, the residents of Antímano were wise to urge caution on Dr. Yonel. They were perfectly willing to admit that street crime was a real threat to everyone, even their new physicians. In the state of Aragua, a Cuban doctor had been murdered in 2003, another killed in the state of Anzoategui in 2004. Several other health workers were killed during the first six years of Barrio Adentro's existence, some while trying to protect their neighbors from armed robbers. At the same time, various stories started circulating about Cubans being spared by criminals when they learned that they were the doctors serving their communities. One doctor related his experience of being threatened in his Caracas barrio by a robber carrying a giant knife, a "cow stabber." When he realized he was about to rob or maim a Cuban doctor, the robber immediately repented, then promised to guide the physician safely past the "real criminals" in the neighborhood. Another more apocryphal tale, which was repeated in the states of Lara and Miranda, and even by those who visited Cuban medical brigades operating in Honduras, tells of thieves who get angry with their victims because they carry no money, and so they want to kill them. But when they learn that their victims are Cuban physicians, they apologize profusely and give them some money, saying they had better have something in their pockets so the next band of robbers doesn't decide to murder them.

We were standing beside two new, shiny white and green dental chairs, made in China and shipped with the dentists from Cuba. Dr. Yonel patted them fondly, but then revealed that he wished for more equipment and materials someday. "I work with one colleague here and we do very basic procedures—fillings, extractions, and other small repairs—because there are thousands of local residents who have gone untreated for years and years, and many of them have never had any dental care at all. So there's no equipment yet for root canals and other more complicated operations—that will simply have to wait."

"There's so many of you, it's like an army of doctors," I said.

"You could say," he said, and grinned, "that we are an army of peace."

The Antímano Health Committees

Immediately after talking with Dr. Yonel, we went to a meeting of health committee representatives from more than forty neighborhoods within the barrio of Antímano. The meeting took place in the largest meeting hall in the area, which happened to be a simple concrete box of a structure, painted yellow, that belonged to an independent Evangelical Pentecostal Church called Comunidad Cristiana: Nueva Vida (New Life Christian Community). The room was spare, the only decoration a bright cloth that hung over a wooden lectern. One of the pastors of the church was wearing jeans and a Che Guevara T-shirt as he leaned against the side wall and listened to speakers. Four sociology students had come from the Central University of Venezuela, a place that has often been depicted as an anti-Chávez institution because of opposition political protests generated there in recent years. It is, however, also home to professors and students who support the Bolivarian Revolution—of these four, two young women wholeheartedly supported Chávez, while the two young men were *ni ni's* ("neither nors"— people who are neither for nor against the president). These two didn't like Chávez's confrontational attitude with the political opposition, but strongly favored all the social programs implemented by the government. All four agreed with their sociology professor that they should do a research project that was of real use to people in the barrios.

The students were offering assistance to health committees that had been compiling, in isolated fashion, all kinds of data about the social and health status of their own particular small neighborhoods. The students offered to create master lists on their computers, as well as to systematize certain questions and data so they would be consistent for every committee. They also offered to compile more reliable data about the condition of dwellings, including the type of construction and amenities in all structures. Eventually they hoped to present the barrio of Antímano with a complete data set on important community issues affecting all of its 250,000 residents.

The audience, made up mostly of women, was delighted with the offer. Some of them were hoping to work alongside the university students, since they had been going back to school to study computer science and social sciences part-time in Mission Sucre classes and wanted to gain the skills to perform their own data collection and analysis. (Mission Sucre is the educational mission that provides part-time, continuing education at the university level.) As the meeting proceeded, committee members brought up other issues, such as the importance of continuing to promote breast-feeding since some young mothers were still being influenced by the heavy advertising for commercial formula. There was a short discussion about birth control, with everyone lauding the free contraception available in various forms at each walk-in clinic and asking for even more information to be provided by both doctors and health committee volunteers. No one, however, brought up the subject of abortion, which generally is not accepted by most lower-class Venezuelan women. For this reason, I was told, the Cuban doctors, who are used to providing abortion on demand in their own country, do not proselytize about the subject to their Venezuelan patients.

One of the women health committee members wanted to point out to the university students that the *entrenadores deportivos,* or "sports trainers," and the large numbers of people who took their exercise classes should not be neglected in the study. "Their activity is making a very significant contribution to the health of our communities," she said. "In fact, the sanctuary of this church is filled every morning with middle-aged adults and grandparents doing their aerobics."

Barrio Adentro Deportivo

In addition to Cuban physicians, many other Cubans aid the Venezuelan people, including nurses, physical rehabilitation specialists, dentists, laboratory technicians, and opticians. On my first trip to Venezuela, I visited four different Barrio Adentro sites in four different Caracas barrios, but never had an opportunity to talk to a family physician. At two places, they were too busy to chat with visitors, at another the doctor was absent because she was taking a three-week vacation in Cuba, and at the fourth stop, I met Dr. Yonel, the young dentist. But it was another professional I met, not a doctor at all, who epitomized the spirit of revolutionary solidarity that Cubans share with the Venezuelan people.

He was a tall, slender black man who appeared beside me at an evening fiesta in one of Caracas's poorest barrios where we were watching eight- and nine-year-olds give a lively dramatic dance performance. He looked as if he could have been a major league pitcher, the kind of guy who might have come on in relief in the ninth inning at Camden Yards in Baltimore and shut down the Orioles. At least he looked that way to the young woman beside me, a baseball fan who had studied briefly in Cuba and attended numerous ball games. She smiled with amazement and pulled a baseball card out of a small collection she kept in her purse. Yes, it really was Felipe Fernandez. Played for the Camaguey team and for the Cuban national team. Was in the top ten of all-time relief pitchers in terms of lifetime saves. Had been with the team the night they beat the Orioles in Baltimore during the summer of 1999. (I had been there, having driven ninety minutes south from my home in Pennsylvania to watch the game with my two young sons. If I remember correctly, the Orioles were so far behind that night that the relief pitchers never appeared.)

As the big barrio crowd danced long into the night, Felipe and I sipped our beer and chatted. I listened to a story that would be totally foreign to almost all the professional athletes that dominate sports in North America, Europe, and much of the rest of the world. This star athlete was nearly forty years old when he retired. He was fit and good-looking. So, what was he doing? Was he making TV ads selling shaving cream or modeling tight-fitting T-shirts?

Not Felipe. He had volunteered to live in a poor, crime-ridden barrio in South America. Minimum contract: a two-year commitment with option to renew. Contract pay: $200 a month. Contract accommodations: a tiny, spare bedroom in the home of a barrio family. Leisure activities: tossing balls to raggedy kids, exploring the city on the Metro, and dancing with his neighbors at neighborhood fiestas.

While Felipe was still playing baseball, he had begun preparing himself for a second career. For several years during the off-season, he enrolled in a rigorous university program for athletic trainers, a profession that emphasizes health and fitness education even more than sports training. When he retired from pitching, he worked briefly as a baseball trainer with the Camaguey team in Cuba's national league, but then he noticed a more challenging opportunity. The Cuban medical teams that were providing care for millions of poor Venezuelans wanted sports trainers to work with them. *Salud integral*, comprehensive health, is holistic health. Health providers are expected to attend to promoting good health just as much as fighting disease and treating sickness.

While Felipe spent some of his afternoons coaching kids in baseball and basketball after school, his primary duties revolved around fitness programs that were coordinated directly with Barrio Adentro clinics. The doctors recommended, even prescribed, participation in the morning aerobics and exercise classes for middle-aged and elderly residents, many of whom had been fighting chronic health problems for years. The detailed lists in each medical office showed that large numbers of the older population were afflicted with hypertension. Though many had suffered from poor nutrition in the past, with increased employment opportunities and subsidized food, many people, young housewives included, were gaining too much weight.

Emphasizing preventive medicine, Felipe and the medical team devised new exercise and nutrition regimens for individuals and families, and enlisted their participation and support for the community-wide efforts to help neighbors whose health risks were most severe. The enthusiasm for physical fitness seemed to be catching on; at the fiesta, a group of *abuelitas* (little grandmothers) who met three or four times a week in Felipe's aerobics classes kept dancing through the night.

At the time, though I was full of admiration for Felipe's individual commitment, I had no idea of the size of the overall Cuban contribution in sports training. I later learned that the first pilot program began in the municipality of Libertador in Caracas in 2002, several months before the first Barrio Adentro doctors arrived. This small group of sixteen sports professors grew to fifty by June 2003; as their numbers multiplied many-fold throughout the country, they became officially known as Barrio Adentro Deportivo (sports inside the neighborhood). By 2004, there were over 5,000 Cuban women and men teaching health and sports, and similar numbers were deployed over the rest of the decade. Many other famous athletes have done their part for international solidarity, such as Ariel, the Olympic champion middleweight boxer who was my son's boxing coach during our stay in the mountains of Lara. He was so modest that we never knew of his true identity until we returned to the United States.[2]

Health Committees Empowering Women

Dr. Maria Hansen, a former university professor and a director of social education projects of PDVSA, told a group meeting in Maracay in 2005, "The health committee is one of the organizations of the base community, where the community can begin acquiring what will become popular power."[3] Sometimes this popular power is expressed by collective groups in openly political ways. In August of 2004, when President Chávez's supporters easily defeated the national recall vote initiated by the political opposition, their favorite political chant was "Ooh, ah, Chávez no se va!" (Chávez won't go). Before the election in the small agricultural state of Yaracuy, 15,000 Chávez supporters, including many members of local health committees, gathered for a last-minute rally where they succinctly and loudly explained why they kept backing the president with their new version of the chant: "Ooh, ah, Barrio no se va!"[4]

On many other occasions, the empowerment gained through participation in the health committees has led to deep personal commitment and transformation. Cuban journalist Enrique Ubieta described the evolution in the consciousness and activity of Rosario, a woman who lives in Nueva Esparta (otherwise known as Isla Margarita, a prime vacation spot). First she became involved in her local health committee, then decided that she and her husband would provide a room in their house for the first Cuban doctor in their neighborhood. Over time, Rosario began volunteering for other duties, working for free at Barrio Adentro in the mornings, and completing her high school course work in Mission Ribas, the educational mission that allows adults to finish their secondary education in the afternoon and evening classes. Finally, she was qualified to take a job as a paid nursing assistant in one of the local walk-in clinics.[5]

The same thing happened with my neighbor Elsy Perez in Monte Carmelo. She had been a member of the original health committee that welcomed the first Cuban doctor and the first dentist to the village in 2004. She gave the doctor a room in her house until permanent quarters could be arranged. Elsy began volunteering regularly at a local ambulatorio, then worked as a practical nurse at the local hospital in nearby Sanare. She also studied intently in the three-year nursing program of Mission Sucre, and in 2009 was completing her thesis, an analysis of local health needs, that was the final step in earning her degree.

With the maturation of Barrio Adentro, some functions that were provided on an ad hoc or volunteer basis have been regularized and formalized. In the case of most community kitchens in the barrios of Caracas, the cooks are still preparing free meals for their poorest and oldest neighbors as long as the local Barrio Adentro doctors judge this is necessary. But now the cooks receive regular salaries for their labor as well as free ingredients to help meet their families' needs. In Monte Carmelo, the development of community council self-government has allowed the village to pay directly for the doctors' meals that were once prepared voluntarily by the health committee. Much of their food is cooked in the same kitchen at the elementary school that now prepares two meals per day for each schoolchild; yet the community council, with its sense of propriety and good accounting, insists on reimbursing the school for the exact amount spent on preparing the doctors' meals. In addition, the community council can now make decisions in concert with the local health committee about large projects, such as the construction and expansion of facilities. In 2009, rather than have to wait for the endless maneuverings of state bureaucracies, the community council decided to use its direct access to federal funds to expand the space in the *ambulatorio* so that it can accommodate both a small laboratory and one more doctor.

The health committees were often the vehicle through which local women began to assert themselves and take an active role in their communities. As with other neighborhood-based participatory groups in the Bolivarian Revolution, the majority of participants are women, and with time more and more of them take leadership roles as the heads of community banking committees and the leaders of community councils. It is quite possible that the participation of Venezuelan women in the health committees is influencing the career choices of their daughters: 73 percent of the students studying in Medicina Integral Comunitaria are female. Also, it can't hurt that a high proportion of the Cuban doctors in Venezuela are women (though the percentage of female medical volunteers does not seem to be published, the Cuban Ministry of Health has recorded that since 1999 more than 50 percent of all Cuban physicians have been female).

Outstanding Examples at the Local Level

In 2007 and 2008, Dr. Edita was the only Venezuelan doctor who worked with the Cubans in the Barrio Adentro program in our area (our village of Monte Carmelo, was located in the large rural municipality (*municipio*) of Andres Eloy Bello, population 50,000, which includes the town of Sanare, population 25,000, and over one hundred hamlets scattered throughout the mountains). The other eleven Venezuelan doctors practicing full-time in the area, were in private practice, five as general practitioners and the other six as specialists. None of these eleven worked at the public hospital, which was staffed by a rotating group of five part-time government-employed doctors who came from outside the area, each of them traveling to the Sanare facility for a few days each week to treat the local populace.[6] Two made the hour-and-a-half drive from the nearest big city of Barquisimeto, and the other three drove farther from the neighboring state of Zulia. Frequently they missed their appointed days and the hospital was desperately in need of an attending physician, especially at nighttime. They called Dr. Edita.

"She's incredible," said Dr. Barbara, the Cuban doctor who worked for nearly two years with Dr. Edita at the Barrio Adentro walk-in clinic in Palo Verde, a village that lies just outside of Sanare. "If she's not here or at the hospital, people will simply go to her home and knock on the door. And, of course, she sees them all."

Dr. Edita had already completed her specialist's training and was working as a pediatrician committed to helping the poor even before the Chávez government came to power. When Barrio Adentro asked for Venezuelan physicians to train in a two-year residency as specialists in comprehensive community medicine, she was one of the first to sign up. She completed the training in 2006 and the following year, when I met her, was sharing an office with Dr. Barbara, who had arrived five months earlier and replaced the previous Cuban doctor. Each doctor had a desk, one on each side of the room, where they received a steady stream of patients while the medical students assigned to work with them performed various tasks. One mother arrived with four little children, two on her knee and two standing and clinging to her. The students moved in and entertained the children one by one, then managed to measure them and examine their eyes, ears, and throats. Meanwhile Dr. Barbara took extensive notes on the medical history of the mother, for she was the one who was ill.

The files on individuals and families are extensive and allow the doctors and students to review the various trends within the community. They use this information to create wall charts describing the predominant health care problems in Palo Verde. This provides them with a comprehensive view of the most pressing local needs that comprehensive community medicine must address. One important component of the medical team's work is educating the public about preventive measures. Many of the common maladies enumerated on the wall charts—such as diabetes, asthma, and hypertension—are combated by introducing exercise programs and changing diets. There are also a variety of informative charts describing public sanitation measures and good nutrition. Posters near the entrances display different kinds of birth control that are available and encourage women to discuss them with their doctors and nurses.

As already discussed, the rapid improvement in the overall health of Venezuelans has mostly been due to the rapid movement toward universal community-based care, rather than any high-tech secrets. Big gains in lowering mortality rates were made in a few years even though big investments at the hospital level of care were just beginning. There are, however, some medium-tech solutions that can be helpful if the community can afford them. For example, our municipality invested in oversized, sturdy Toyota jeeps for its Campo Adentro program, which takes Barrio Adentro into the countryside. The jeeps can transport medical teams of ten or twelve doctors and students into the sparsely populated, remote parts of the municipality. Since they can make two- to five- hour trips over muddy, rutted roads that are impassable for other cars, the big Toyotas also double as emergency vehicles that can bring patients out of the *campo* in case of life-threatening situations. The most telling local statistic related to this service, according to Mayor Orozco, was that in the first eight months of 2007, for the first time ever, not a single mother or child in the entire area lost their lives during childbirth.

7. New Doctors for Venezuela

The best way of telling is doing.

—JOSÉ MARTÍ

On August 19, 1960, Che Guevara spoke to the Cuban militia about organizing "public health so as to provide treatment for the greatest possible number of people." He explained that the practice of revolutionary medicine would be a vocation based on public service and revolutionary doctors would define themselves by their practice of solidarity and equality. He finished with his favorite quotation from José Martí: *Hacer es la mejor manera de decir*—"The best way of telling is doing."

The Cuban doctors working with Barrio Adentro are following in the spirit of Martí's maxim: they are teaching by doing. In January of 2006, less than three years after they launched the ambitious public health program, these physicians began training the first-year medical students who would one day serve as their replacements. In addition to delivering primary health care to the majority of the Venezuelan population, the Cubans have taken on the duties of professor/tutors— working alongside students every day, tutoring them in the skills of recognizing how normal bodies function and diagnosing the abnormalities that are signs of disease, and giving them formal lectures in medical science. They are demonstrating, by their comportment and attention to preventive health care in the barrios, how a revolutionary doctor promotes trust among his or her patients and the community, and then involves them in creating a healthier society.

In January of 2007, I visited the town of Sanare in the state of Lara with a group of of U.S. college students and took them to the newly built Barrio Adentro II Diagnostic Center. It serves the municipality of Andres Eloy Blanco, which is composed of 25,000 residents in Sanare, the main agricultural town, and another 25,000 populating more than one hundred villages and hamlets spread over rugged mountainous terrain. One of those villages is Monte Carmelo, where I took up residence eight months later.

We were able to spend a few hours discussing the new health care programs with two Cuban ophthalmologists, Dr. Frank and his young colleague, Dr. Eulogio, who worked with patients at the Diagnostic Center who were referred to them by all the Barrio Adentro I primary care offices in the area. But they also had another job—training the doctors who will one day replace them. In 2007, there were forty-two local residents of the municipality in the first and second year of the intensive medical training program known as Medicina Integral Communitaria; in Venezuela everyone refers to the program by its acronym, MIC. Near the end of our meeting, Dr. Frank introduced us to four medical students, ranging from twenty to twenty-six years old, and one fellow who was much older. "I'm forty-seven years old," he said, "but I'm determined to finish all six years of study then do my residency. I've always been interested in medicine and spent more than fifteen years assisting a physician in his office, but I never dreamed it was possible for me to go to university and become a doctor."

Juan and the other three students did not attend the traditional established university in the big city of Barquisimeto an hour and a half away. Instead, a new university had come to them. The students were spending the morning at the side of Dr. Frank as he made his rounds. They observed diagnoses and care and discussed the physiology and pathology pertinent to their current studies. The doctor said he kept track of the subject matter the students were studying each week in their classes so that he could demonstrate appropriate procedures or anatomical lessons. "Sometimes it's exceedingly simple," he explained, "if they are studying the pulmonary system and the pathologies of the lung, then first of all they ought to know what a variety of healthy lungs sound like. So when I'm listening with my stethoscope to someone's perfectly healthy lungs, I make sure the students get to listen and ask questions about what they are hearing."

After studying for six years, then completing a two-year residency in comprehensive community medicine, the MIC students will become part of the corps of the full-fledged family physicians who will staff Barrio Adentro offices in this area and other parts of the nation. The commitment required on the part of the students, most of them low-income campesinos, requires long-term effort and support. Although the education is free, and the students receive modest stipends to help with their living expenses while completing their studies, Juan wanted me to understand the importance of family: "The only reason I can pursue a medical career is the support I get, both financial and moral, from my wife, her family, and my parents and brothers."

Dr. Frank and Dr. Eulogio emphasized that their Venezuelan students were the beneficiaries of a "revolution within the revolution" in Cuba, where many systems of education have been radically changing since 2000. For example, in 2004 Cuban medical students began going on rounds to see patients in their first year, as in Venezuela, rather than waiting until the fourth year as in the past. Other kinds of progress, having nothing directly to do with medicine, are also evident in the educational revolution in Cuba. For instance, there is an emphasis on increasing the quality of primary and secondary schools and training more teachers, so that class sizes, already reduced to twenty students or less, will not exceed fifteen in the future.

Although they thought the scholastic achievement of their Venezuelan students was impressive, the Cuban ophthalmologists emphasized something else: "What is even more satisfying for us to see is the creation of moral and ethical values that allow them to really influence their own communities." From their experience in Cuba they think that the social consciousness and emotional maturity required for the job is at least as important as having an advanced aptitude for studying science. In Cuba, the selection process has changed from one that used to favor only the students who scored high marks on academic tests, since it was found that those people did not always make the most conscientious doctors. There is, of course, still emphasis on having ability in science, but equal weight is given to the student's potential for working with colleagues and communities, and understanding and sympathizing with all kinds of patients.

"I think we and our students are creating a new model of what a medical professional is supposed to be," explained Dr. Eulogio. "The old Venezuelan stereotype of a doctor, at least in the cities, was somebody driving around in a fancy car with black windows and air-conditioning. So nobody knows who they are—people only get to see them in their offices if they can pay."

How MIC Was Created

When the Barrio Adentro system of primary health was getting started in Venezuela, the number of Cuban doctors working in the system multiplied at an astonishing rate, from fifty-three in the Liberator district of Caracas in April of 2003, to more than 10,000 by May of 2004. During this time, Cuban and Venezuelan medical educators who were involved with Barrio Adentro were also contemplating the best way to incorporate Venezuelan doctors into the program.

Dr. Juan Carlos Marcano, who worked with the Health Ministry as a Barrio Adentro coordinator in those years, told a reporter that they were having trouble recruiting existing Venezuelan doctors or the medical students who were passing through the traditional, elite university system. "Most students are studying to earn money," he said, "changing the culture of established medical schools will be difficult."[1] The majority of Venezuelan doctors, he felt, were still going to be attracted to practicing high-priced specialties in private practice in wealthier neighborhoods.

There was also discussion about eventually expanding medical education as part of an effort to open higher education to working-class and poor students within the newly chartered Bolivarian University of Venezuela (Universidad Bolivariana de Venezuela, or UBV) and at a few other experimental universities in other parts of the country. Another idea, floated by Minister of Education Hector Navarro, was to create a three-year crash course that would create a kind of para-physician, competent in certain emergency surgical and life-saving situations, thus taking some of the burden off of full-fledged physicians. This idea never took off.

In the fall of 2003, young Cuban medical graduates arrived to work side by side in Barrio Adentro with their older, experienced compatriots who had started the program that spring and summer. These young doctors, like almost every aspiring Cuban graduate, were required to complete their specialty by doing a two-year residency in a primary health facility. Dr. Radames Borroto, director of the National School of Public Health in Havana and the National Academic Coordinator for Barrio Adentro in Caracas, explained to Cuban journalist Enrique Ubieta that the Cubans "who finished their training here have had an extraordinary preparation, because they have had an assisting practice that is very much superior to what they could have had in Cuba."[2] Borroto said this was the moment that the idea of training Venezuelans was born, because "in many states simultaneously many people were coming forward and asking to work alongside our doctors."

Some of the Venezuelans were students from the elite universities, such as a young, revolutionary-minded graduate named Joel Pantoja, age twenty-six, who had just graduated from medical school at the University of Carabobo in Valencia. He and other young colleagues wanted to set up their own Barrio Adentro Clinic because their local state and city governments were led by anti-Chávistas who flatly rejected any help from Cuban doctors.[3] The Venezuelan and Cuban governments decided that recent Venezuelan medical graduates like Dr. Pantoja could join the young Cuban residents working in Barrio Adentro, thus becoming the first Venezuelan doctors to complete the new residency training. As soon as the residency program was institutionalized in early 2004, Venezuelan doctors who wanted to serve poor communities had a means to prepare themselves. By 2006, there was a group of 1,013 Venezuelans who successfully completed their residencies and became full-fledged Barrio Adentro practitioners.

In addition to this group, several hundred Venezuelan students were attending ELAM, the Latin American School of Medicine in Havana, who would be graduating between 2005 and 2008. Eventually they formed "Batallion 51," a special group of volunteers who were willing to serve Barrio Adentro in the most inaccessible and primitive locations in the country. All in all, however, these new recruits were not sufficient to meet the public health needs of the nation, for the Chávez government was estimating the need for a veritable army of physicians, twenty to thirty thousand strong, to staff the four levels of care that would eventually be created within Barrio Adentro. While the residency programs would only produce a small fraction of the Venezuelan doctors needed for Barrio Adentro, it led to the creation of Medicina Integral Comunitaria by a team of Venezuelan and Cuban medical educators who were planning an entire new system of medical education. Dr. José Jean Carlos Yepez, the Venezuelan who is often credited with being the "father of MIC,"[4] was vice rector of the Colegio Universitario Francisco de Miranda, an experimental university in the state of Falcon. In 2003 he was named chairman of a national commission to develop and oversee the National Training Program in Comprehensive Community Medicine. The commission brought together members from the health ministry and six Venezuelan universities with a team of six Cuban medical educators who were experienced in both the development of Barrio Adentro and the curriculum for the new University Polyclinic physician training program in Cuba.

Dr. Yepez and some of the other Venezuelan representatives were already involved in the planning for one of the large educational missions of the Chávez government, Mission Sucre. It was created to bring university-level education directly to poor and working-class citizens in the barrios and rural towns, thus providing a local "university without walls" that maximized community participation. The Venezuelan and Cuban medical educators on the commission decided to utilize Mission Sucre to recruit students who would then be trained in conjunction with Barrio Adentro.

In order to teach medicine in the barrios and towns of almost all 335 municipalities of Venezuela, it was necessary to incorporate a large percentage of the Cuban doctors working in Barrio Adentro. The Cubans were fortunate to have a new medical curriculum at their disposal that had just been developed for the general medicine program in the Cuban polyclinic medical schools in 2004 (University Polyclinic Medical Training Program). This curriculum was ideal for adaptation to the needs of MIC in Venezuela because it was designed to be incorporated into a community-based settings just like Mission Sucre.

MIC Structure

Both the University Polyclinic Medical Training Program and the MIC program differ from the traditional model of medical education developed in the United States in the early twentieth century that strongly influenced university medical programs in Cuba, Venezuela, and many other countries. In 1910 educational innovator Abraham Flexner wrote a report for the Rockefeller Foundation that helped systematize a four-year term of medical study and more rigorous scientific training within authorized university-based medical schools in the United States. The Flexnerian model became standardized throughout the United States and much of the world, either in four-year or six-year programs. Students spend their first years studying separate basic sciences (physiology, anatomy, etc.), and in later years move on to the clinical sciences. Finally they are exposed to practice in real medical situations in a hospital setting.

The medical schools of the polyclinic program in Cuba and MIC in Venezuela dispense with the traditional university and its associated teaching hospital, even though they still offer classroom instruction in scientific medicine. From the beginning of the first year, this class-room education is supplemented with a great deal of participation and observation with family medicine specialists as they attend to patients in nearby Barrio Adentro offices and diagnostic centers. In the sites in Venezuela I visited, small groups of students typically work four hours each morning with a Cuban physician/teacher at a small Barrio Adentro consulting office or the larger, more modern diagnostic center. At times the students may work at the Barrio Adentro site in their own specific neighborhoods, but they also rotate to other nearby locales to experience working in several settings with various experienced personnel.

In the afternoons, students converge on a central location devoted to classroom education, and are taught by many of the same doctors who are their tutors during the mornings. If they do not have a class at a particular hour, they make use of computer resources and a library of written reference material, and organize group study sessions among themselves.

The highly organized classroom material involves a sophisticated curriculum that was prepared by sixty medical professors in Cuba who were specialists in a broad range of the biomedical and socio-medical sciences. The core of traditional scientific subject matter that Flexner identified a century ago is still maintained, but it is not taught in distinct courses in separate disciplines. The new curriculum devised by the Cubans, now used in all of their medical schools, combines these separate subjects into new interdisciplinary courses. One of these is a four-part, first- and second-year course known as morphophysiology, which weaves together such courses as anatomy, physiology, genetics, cellular and molecular biology, and immunology. Another major interdisciplinary course is morphophysiopathology, studied in the second year; it combines the other sciences related to clinical practice; for example, clinical laboratory, imaging, parasitology, microbiology, and anatomic pathology, as well as the main immune, hemodynamic, genetic and neoplastic pathological processes.[5] Highly developed DVD materials have been compiled for each course, so that every class lecture is accompanied by a specific DVD that is used intermittently by the professor during the lecture; all students have their own copies of these DVDs for further study and review.

The Latin American School of Medicine in Havana still maintains a separate campus for international students and has some curricular features that differ from both the MIC program and the Cuban Polyclinic University program. However, ELAM has adopted the same interdisciplinary courses that the other medical programs use. Dr. Juan Carrizo, director of ELAM, described the positive aspects of the scientific curriculum in a discussion with medical education innovators from Canada, Australia, Venezuela, and the Philippines:

> We have replaced the teaching of sciences in isolation—anatomy one semester, microbiology the next—with a morphophysiological pedagogical approach, which enables students to better analyze, problem-solve and integrate knowledge in a cumulative, comprehensive way. We design our courses so that everything is connected, making it easier to understand the patient as a whole, while being careful not to compromise the quality of the students' scientific training. We have found that students absorb scientific knowledge better with this methodology and are better prepared to solve clinical health problems, pursue research and develop professionally.[6]

Cuban medical professionals who have worked in Venezuela are convinced that the interdisciplinary courses work best within community-based programs like MIC. Dr. Barbara, who let me observe her daily routine of working in the Barrio Adentro office with MIC students, feels that the MIC education system is a significant improvement on the older Cuban model, and not just because of the social experience that integrates the students' studies with their work and their communities. She thinks they are learning faster, that the combination of on-site participation and observation with demanding classroom instruction enables them to assimilate the information more quickly and ask more pertinent questions. When I asked if she thought the daily work component was too much of a distraction from the business of regular study for her students, she laughed and answered, "On the contrary. Their excitement about their academic learning, combined with their enthusiasm for interacting with and understanding our patients, makes them ask questions all the time, so that they have a much more dynamic experience than students have in conventional universities in Cuba, and this accelerates the learning process. I think by the time they get into their third year, they are at least a year further advanced than traditional Cuban students. They seem more like trusted medical colleagues than students."

Dr. Borroto, who led the formal evaluation of the first three years of MIC training throughout Venezuela, confirmed this opinion in an interview: "The result, I tell you, is the same level as in Cuba, in content, in assimilation of the content, and when you look at the appropriation of knowledge, it is superior to Cuba."[7] One reason he thinks this is true is that the Venezuelan context is truly fresh and disconnected from the old teaching methods. When integral teaching of multidisciplinary subjects was first introduced in Cuba, it incorporated more student practice at the polyclinics and neighborhood consulting offices, but the medical faculty was not necessarily ready to change their approach to teaching science. "They merely wanted to transport the old 'Ciencias Basicas' to the policlinico," explained Dr. Borroto.[8] The conception of a new system that uses modern technology and communication, computers, DVDs, CDs, and videos to transform the study of basic sciences into something new was resisted for a while in Cuba. But because these curricular advances were fully incorporated into the MIC program in Venezuela, Cuban doctors who have been exposed to them are able to return home and facilitate the use of the new methods in polyclinic settings.

The MIC Curriculum

The following is a brief summary of the MIC curriculum describing the course work, clinical study, and internship requirements that are fulfilled in each of the six years required to complete the degree in *Medicina Integral Comunitaria*, or Comprehensive Community Medicine.[9]

Year one is dominated by lectures in Human Morphophysiology—this is the interdisciplinary combination of all the basic sciences that were taught separately in the traditional Flexnerian medical school. There is also a Community Health and Medicine component (social-medical sciences and social sciences) that includes introduction to social sciences, introduction to primary health care, social communication, and civics.

Year two continues the study of basic sciences in Human Morphophysiology and begins the study of Human Morphophysiopathology; the Community Health and Medicine component covers public health, history of health, epidemiology and hygiene, medical research, community intervention and health analysis, and an introduction to Latin American political thought.

Year three places more scientific emphasis on clinical medicine, and includes courses in pharmacology I and II, and the psychology of health care; Community Health and Medicine covers the same subjects as in year two, plus a course in medical ethics.

Year four concentrates on Clinical Medicine once again and includes Pediatrics I and II, Psychiatry, and Obstetrics and Gynecology I. The Community Health and Medicine component includes normal growth and development, family health, care of oncology patients, community health analysis, community rehabilitation, and special environments.

Year five moves into the internship phase of Clinical Medicine and concentrates on General Surgery; Orthopedics, Traumatology and Rehabilitation; Pediatrics III: Hospital Care; Obstetrics and Gynecology II: Hospital Care; Urology, Dermatology, Otolaryngology, and Ophthalmology. The Community Health and Medicine areas are public health, administration, disaster medicine, forensics, toxicology, principles of medical research, and the study of natural and traditional medicine.

Year six emphasizes the internship in Medicina Integral Comunitaria; students work on three rotations of twelve weeks each in Adult Care, Children's Care, Care of Women and Pregnancy, and one rotation of nine weeks in Surgical Care.

The Rapid Growth of
Medicina Integral Comunitaria in Venezuela

There were those who thought that Fidel Castro was dreaming the impossible when he spoke to the first 1,500 graduates of ELAM in 2005. He said that Cuba would begin training 100,000 new doctors who would serve the poor and marginalized populations of the world's developing countries. And, he claimed, the task would be accomplished in only ten years!

In revolutionary Latin America, this quixotic optimism is shared by others. Che Guevara once wrote his mother that he could feel the "ribs of Rocinante [Don Quixote's horse] under his heels" as he was about to take off on another adventure.

Hugo Chávez has often joked about his own quixotic tendencies, and the political opposition has often accused him of tilting at windmills when he proposed ambitious goals for the nation. His government's response in 2004 was to distribute a million copies of *Don Quixote* free of charge to the Venezuelan people so they could be familiar with this seminal work of Spanish literature. In 2005 the Venezuelan president appeared at Fidel's side and had no hesitation about joining the ludicrously ambitious project: the two small nations vowed to produce 100,000 doctors.

Of this number, they committed themselves to educate 30,000 doctors in family medicine in Venezuela, with the goal being that within ten years, that is, by 2015, they would be ready to take over the operation of Barrio Adentro from the Cubans. Just four years later, while speaking to the nation on his *Alo Presidente* TV show, President Chávez indicated that this ambitious goal had every chance of being achieved. He announced that the current enrollment in MIC was 24,811. Of these, 8,875 students were finishing their fourth year; 7,819 completing the third; 3,513 the second; and 4,604 the first. This did not include the approximately 5,000 students who were enrolled in premedical studies and would begin the first year of MIC in 2010. Chávez declared that *un ejército de batas blancas*, "an army in white jackets," would go into battle in 2010 in Barrio Adentro clinics and hospitals all over the country, and help win the struggle to install a new universal public medical system. He was referring to those 8,875 students, wearing their white cotton doctors' coats, who after finishing their the fourth year of MIC were ready to assume their internships alongside the approximately 14,000 Cuban and Venezuelan physicians who were already working at all the different levels of Barrio Adentro.

Obviously, an account written in 2010 cannot guarantee that all these physicians in training will be usefully employed five years in the future. But it can, at the least, cite some studies by Cuban and Venezuelan researchers that indicate that Medicina Integral Comunitaria is headed in the right direction. Research published in 2008 showed that the dropout rate was rather high during the first two years the MIC program was in existence; in 2006 and 2007, 4,503, or 26 percent of all students, dropped out, mainly due to poor academic performance. This retention or pass rate of 74 percent improved as initial shortcomings of the MIC program were rapidly overcome. During the following academic year the pass rate rose to 82 percent for first-year students and 94 percent for second-year students.[10] One might safely assume (although no data are available at this time) that the passing rate kept increasing as students completed their third- and fourth-year studies, since the students had already proven their mettle and become more and more dedicated to their medical vocation. With more students enrolled in 2009 and 2010, it appeared that even with some attrition among the newcomers, there would be 30,000 students graduating with MIC degrees between 2012 and 2017.

The medical directors of MIC have demonstrated they are not simply interested in collecting impressive numbers as they push the students through the demanding six-year curriculum. They also intend to improve the program as it keeps growing. In March 2008, when I entered a walk-in clinic in Palo Verde near Sanare for a scheduled conversation with medical students, the health committee member who was serving as receptionist informed me that everyone had rushed to Sanare. There was an "emergency meeting" of all Barrio

Adentro staff and medical students in the area. The emergency, I found out later, was an an action research study being conducted by the National Academic Coordinating Committee of Barrio Adentro, which was making an intensive tour of the country to conduct interviews with the students and professors who work together in MIC. In two months these investigators managed to interview a sizable cross section of the whole MIC program, 1,277 faculty and 2,594 students. By August 2008, they had reviewed the data and identified the major challenges ahead:

1. Doing a better job at student selection and retention, thus making it easier for the primarily low-income and marginalized student population to overcome obstacles and succeed.

2. Assuring the best assimilation of new pedagogical concepts on the part of the Cuban family medicine specialists since they are required to make an extra effort organizationally, academically, and individually with new courses that are quite different from those they studied as medical students.

3. Dealing with the fact that Barrio Adentro itself is being expanded and adapted as part of a new national health system, and has had uneven development in different parts of the country. That is, the level of participation of local communities and the support given to local students of medicine could vary widely.

4. Meeting the growing demands by communities and patients who, after five years of Barrio Adentro service, have new and much higher expectations of what constitutes good care.

Dr. Borroto, who played an important role both in developing the MIC program and working with the National Academic Coordinating Committee in preparing this evaluation on progress to date, was careful to add a cautionary note: "Any final measure of the program's success—its impact on health services and accessibility, on the health status of the population, and on the graduates' future commitment to a career in public service—is still several years away."[11]

Other Important Gains from the MIC Program

The Venezuelans gain immensely from the MIC program because they will be able to staff a universal primary health care system with their own personnel in the near future, but they are not the only ones who benefit from this revolutionary form of medical education. As a result of collaborating and improvising during the evolution of Medicina Integral Comunitaria Cubans have managed to develop whole new areas of expertise. For the more experienced Cuban doctors, including those who were well established in their specialties and had worked abroad in the past, there were new kinds of educational gains. Dr. Borroto and his team of public health researchers have emphasized that most Cuban doctors who teach in Venezuela have had to constantly update their own professional training in order to keep up with the demanding course work of their MIC students. Of the approximately 13,000 Cuban physicians who were working in Venezuela in 2008 in various capacities, about half also served as teachers of comprehensive community medicine in the MIC program, and most of them had had to complete more academic study in order to fulfill their teaching duties.

According to a report in *MEDICC Review,* in 2008 "A total of 6,715 faculty—primary care specialists who also staff Barrio Adentro clinics—teach in the program; 4,602 (68.5%) of them have attained the academic rank of at least Instructor or Assistant Professor, having met requirements established by Cuba's Ministry of Higher Education." Often their advanced study involved a combination of courses in Cuba, seminars with other doctors serving in Venezuela, and a variety of computer-based extension courses that could be completed online. For those who were asked to manage the complexities at the state and municipality levels, an eighteen- to twenty-four-month master's program in medical education was offered through

Cuba's National School of Public Health; 126 faculty and program directors working at various levels in Venezuela had obtained these MS degrees.[12]

All of the Cuban doctors who participate in the combination of Barrio Adentro/MIC activities are taking on the difficult task of serving as tutors and professors as well as family physicians. This entails simultaneous attention to practicing medicine, educating the community, communicating with inexperienced colleagues, and teaching at the same time. And the formal teaching with a new curriculum requires extra learning—returning to Cuba for classes, going to seminars with other medical personnel in Venezuela, and completing correspondence courses on the computer. For Cuban physicians, according to journalist and philosopher Enrique Ubieta Gómez, "the most difficult task is becoming teachers. They have to return to school, but the day is full of tasks—consultations, home visits, the tutorial role with students, giving classes at Mission Sucre, taking postgrad and master's classes themselves."[13]

To develop a new kind of medical education in Venezuela, the Cuban doctors have had to take on the task of their own self-development. They have managed to become "six-star doctors," in addition to having achieved "five-star" status, which in itself is fairly rare in medical practice around the world. The "five-star doctor," a concept developed by Dr. Charles Boelen at the World Health Organization, refers to the physician who is ideal for meeting the needs of universal, community-based health programs. The Cuban doctors, most of whom trained as family doctors before specializing in anything else, had the five attributes that Boelen said were required: 1) caregiver; 2) decision maker; 3) communicator; 4) manager; and 5) community leader.

In Venezuela they have added a sixth star: teacher.[14]

The younger Cuban doctors, who graduated from medical school in the first decade of this century and were able to complete their residencies in comprehensive general medicine in Venezuela, were able to expand their medical expertise in a different fashion. They encountered a range of experiences with diseases and maladies that they never would have encountered in Cuba, which will serve as good preparation for other international missions, including future ventures in medical education in other poor and developing countries. There was a similar experience for another group of young Cuban graduates, those who had finished their dentistry programs at Cuban universities and came to Venezuela to complete two-year residencies in Comprehensive General Dentistry (known at home as Estomatologia General Integral, EGI) as they worked in Barrio Adentro dental offices.

The specialty in comprehensive dentistry had been developed ten years earlier in Cuba but had generated little interest there, partly because, according to Dr. Borroto, an attitude among many dentists in Cuba led them to dismiss the value of delivering basic dental services and education at the community level. This may have been because Cuban dentists, as opposed to doctors of comprehensive community medicine, had seldom participated in missions abroad and lacked an appreciation of the extreme needs and lack of care in other countries. In any case, of the 2,900 Cuban dentists who went to Venezuela to serve in Barrio Adentro, three-quarters were young practitioners who served the residency in the EGI specialty. Dr. Borroto felt that this was a "revolutionary" development because the dentists began to return to Cuba with "a kind of training that is much superior and much more pertinent to the health needs of our country."[15] An added benefit of this comprehensive dentistry residency training was that it was open to graduates of Venezuelan dentistry schools too, with the result that more than 2,000 Venezuelan dentists ended up working alongside Cubans in Barrio Adentro. However, the dentistry education program in Venezuela did not expand to offer a full six-year university course of the kind that MIC was offering to prospective physicians.

The medical expertise gained by Cubans in Venezuela was certain to help them on their future international missions, but there is another way, a bit harder to define, that the experience has benefited them. Enrique Ubieta Gómez feels that the Cuban doctors' exposure to the social transformations taking place in South America helps acquaint them with their own history. "In Venezuela and now in Bolivia, there is the added possibility for Cubans to have a reunion with the revolutionary past of their own country, which the immense majority of them did not experience."[16]

This experience of "recycling the revolution," according to Ubieta Gómez, has been part of a general rejuvenation of the internationalist and revolutionary spirit in Cuba that began with the Cuban medical missions to central America and Haiti in 1998. He believes this rejuvenation of Cuban society is the most valuable benefit gained from Cuba's growing cooperation with Venezuela and other ALBA nations, even more valuable than the substantial gains made by exchanging health care services for cheap Venezuelan oil.

This revived internationalist spirit is contagious, for the Cuban doctors have been inspiring role models for their students and the communities they serve. The MIC educational structure allows students to form strong bonds with the doctors who are, in effect, not only tutors sharing their knowledge but also master craftsmen patiently pointing out details and necessary skills to their apprentices. Just as important, they serve as models of humanitarian dedication, transmitting their socialist values by example rather than by proselytizing. Dr. Barbara, who I observed working with patients and students in her Barrio Adentro office, completed other medical missions in Yemen, Ethiopia, and Haiti before coming to Venezuela. She clearly inspired her MIC students from Sanare and Monte Carmelo with her energy and sense of adventure, and now some of these campesinos dream of following in her footsteps and one day volunteering for foreign missions of their own.

8. Building Community Medicine on a Daily Basis

I was born a socialist, so this is the right way for me to finish out my life. Serving the people.

—JOSÉ, 71, first-year student in MIC

Two or three times a week during my year in Venezuela, I would climb the mountainside above Monte Carmelo to visit the cooperative organic farm located on the slopes just below the cloud forest. One day as I made my way up the steep road, a motorcycle came roaring around a deeply rutted curve and disappeared down the mountain in a cloud of dust. I stopped to catch my breath and chat with the farmer who stood by the barbed wire fence next to two of his ten cows. "He's off to class in Sanare," he said as we watched the motorcycle reappear on the paved road far below. "Jonás is only in his second year and already he sees patients."

He was intensely proud that his son was studying to be a medical doctor. So proud that on the following Sunday, when they invited me over to their house, he said once again, "In his second year, he's seeing patients already."

"Remember, Papá," Jonás interrupted, "even though we see the patients and talk to them, we don't make any treatment decisions. We're just there to observe and assist our teachers and ask questions."

"I know that," his father said. "What I mean is that it's important that all of you are learning to talk to the patients, treating them like fellow human beings. Letting them know they can trust you." Then he explained to me why this was so important. His son was not the first person in their extended family to attend medical school. There was a cousin who many years earlier dreamed of being a doctor, and her mother, who was very poor, worked constantly to save every spare coin and told her daughter to study hard. Many family members and friends pitched in to assist the mother in various ways.

"And so the daughter, my cousin, really did manage to go to medical school," explained Jonás's father, "at the big university in the city. It was extremely rare for any campesino to go to university in those days. Then she went on to finish her training in her specialty, and now she lives in Caracas and sees patients in her fancy neighborhood. Of course, as far as she's concerned, I don't exist. None of us exists. She doesn't associate with anyone in the family and won't talk to any of us." Jonás and his father had invited me to join their family and seven other second- and third-year students of MIC for a little rest and relaxation. They had a rare bit of free time for music and dancing, sitting and chatting, and enjoying the view over the valley below. Dr. Barbara, one of the Cuban physicians who held the MIC students to a rigorous schedule the other six days of the week, was taking charge of the family kitchen and learning, with some advice from her students, how to prepare a big pot of the local *sancocho*, a tasty meat-and-vegetable stew that campesinos often eat on festive occasions.

Jonás had graduated from *liceo*, high school, before the MIC medical program began. During the early years of the Bolivarian Revolution, he and other students ventured into isolated hamlets as literacy volunteers, teaching adults to read and urging them to continue in Mission Robinson and complete the equivalent of primary schooling. During this period, Jonás also continued helping his father with the cows, worked with the neighbors when they brought in a harvest, and helped build a modest concrete block house for the family with the support of an interest-free loan from the government.

The group of eight students at Jonás's house told me that their pre-medical year and first year of medical classes were demanding enough to sort out the unmotivated from the serious students who truly feel a vocation in medicine. Jonás and Luisa, who grew up on farms, thought that students like themselves were more likely to stick with the program since they had been accustomed to hard work ever since child-hood. Luisa grew up in La Bucarita, a coffee-growing village on the far side of the municipality, three hours from the main town of Sanare. She had to move in with an elderly relative in Sanare to attend MIC classes, and although she missed the company of her large extended family, she said, "They keep encouraging me, so I'm determined to complete my medical studies." Luisa wanted to return to La Bucarita and become its first full-time doctor. Jonás said he hoped that someday he could travel to remote areas of other nations and serve as an internationalist physician.

Although Sundays were supposedly days of rest and study for the students, they sometimes devoted this day to visiting residents of the Yacambú, who hardly ever saw a doctor. In this lush and deeply forested area, there are over a hundred small hamlets that are much smaller and poorer than La Bucarita and Monte Carmelo, inhabited almost entirely by impoverished coffee farmers. It takes four to six hours to reach some of these places, even if one has a jeep that can negotiate the muddy tracks and overflowing streams in the cloud forest. In the rainy season, the mayor's office would make one of its oversized four-wheel-drive "Campo Adentro" vehicles available, and the Cuban doctors and their students would pack the vehicle with medical and dental supplies and offer one-day mini-clinics. But at other times when the roads were passable, they might venture out with José, a fellow student who owned an old car and knew his way around the obscure routes throughout the Yacambú.

José, a first-year student from Sanare, was seventy-one. Once, his fellow students told me, nearly fifty years ago, he had been a supporter of the revolutionary guerrillas and carried supplies to them in their hideouts in the mountains. The younger students said they were proud of José because, in spite of his age, he worked as hard as anyone at his studies. Some of the other students were nineteen or twenty years old, recently graduated from high school, others were young mothers in their late twenties, a few in their thirties and forties.

"We all have a high level of commitment," said Hilario, a third-year student, "but you have to really admire the women in particular. Many are mothers and have young children and family duties that they have to attend to. Frankly, I don't know how they do it." Hilario was no slouch himself, since at forty-three he could have felt worn out by a lifetime of work at a wide range of jobs including truck driver, carpenter, and construction site manager. "Of course," he pointed out, "few of us students could survive without the help of our families. They encourage us and they support us. We all have somebody who is helping with the expenses."

Each student receives a modest monthly stipend from the government, and while this might be enough money for single people living at home with their parents, it is not nearly enough for those who have families of their own. "Many members of the extended family help with financial support, but the grandparents are the key," said Dilbex, a young mother from Sanare. "Knowing that they are taking good care of the kids makes it possible for me to devote my attention to my studies."

Practicing and Studying Medicine

The physicians in training spent their mornings working with doctors in Sanare or the villages that had their own walk-in clinics, and then switched over to concentrating on demanding academic material in the afternoons. For formal classes, they converged on a central location in Sanare, lugging big, fat three-ring binders stuffed with 400 to 500 sheets of photocopied textbook pages and articles. In their classroom area, there was supplementary material available in books and on the computers, so that during the times when students did not have class they were poring over this material and discussing it with each other.

Magaly and Dilbex told me that the material had become progressively more challenging over the three years they had been studying. During the afternoon lectures by the Cuban doctors, they took copious notes. "Then, in the early evening," they said, "groups of us often meet together, so we can quiz each other after classes." Their notes were backed up by one of the key resources of the MIC program, the DVD material that accompanies each class. While most first- and second-year students cannot afford their own personal computers, someone in their extended families usually had a DVD player so they could review the medical lessons as many times as needed at home. And since students were continually encouraging and helping one another, a student who did not have the equipment for watching the DVDs would be invited to review them in the company of others. Obviously, families had to cooperate, too, for they were willing to give up some television time in order to further the studies of the medical students.

According to Milena and Mariela, also third-year students, the MIC program was more difficult when they began in 2006. "We were the pioneers in that first year, when many of the course materials were still in the process of development. Often we watched older movies or VHS videotapes that were shown on classroom TVs. But there were no extra copies, and in any case, no one around here had VHS machines at home. Even when the first DVDs arrived, things were difficult, because they were a certain kind of disc that we couldn't copy. But now that's all been rectified, and the first- and second-year students have it easy."

These two women had begun studying three and a half years earlier as part of the first MIC class in the municipality. They responded to public announcements that invited interested people to meet with officials at the local Mission Sucre offices, which have charge of all *extra muro* university-level education programs. Mariela, who had recently finished her *bachelerato* (the equivalent of a high school degree), said she had always dreamed of being a doctor, but had doubted she would ever have the opportunity to study at one of the big city universities. "So, when I heard that we might be able to qualify to enter the program in Medicina Integral Comunitaria, I raced down the mountain into Sanare to sign up."

Milena was already married and the mother of a two-year-old daughter when she was accepted into the program, feeling fortunate that she was encouraged by both her husband and his family. By the time I was living in Monte Carmelo, her daughter was five or six, and I would often see her being walked down the road to kindergarten at 8:15 in the morning by her father or her grandfather because Milena was already working at Barrio Adentro. When she and Mariela were accepted into the medical program, they first had to pass the premedical course that was designed to get all students, those fresh out of high school and those who had not attended classes for a long time, performing at the same level.

When they entered the third year of MIC, they received special rewards for their efforts from the government: new laptop computers. This allowed them to study course DVDs, digitalized films and medical articles, and search the medical websites whenever they wanted. They were delighted because they felt that the complexity and intensity of their work had increased in the third year. Specifically, they mentioned their pharmacology course, since it demanded extensive memorization of various chemical compounds and drugs, plus knowledge of dosages and possible side effects on the patient. Third-year students also had special duties to perform in addition to working alongside their Cuban tutors every day. Once every fourteen nights, two of the twenty-eight third-year students were required to stay all night at the CDI, the large modern diagnostic center in the middle of Sanare that opened in 2006. From 8 p.m. to 8 a.m., they helped admit emergency patients and assist the lone Cuban doctor who was on call.

"This is a pretty tough regimen," I said, but Mariela and Milena just smiled and shrugged, as if to say this was what they expected all along.

So then I asked, "How many of the third-year students have dropped out along the way?"

"Five out of thirty-nine are no longer with us. There was only one who thought it was simply too hard, too much work. Another is having a baby and hopes she can return. Three others felt the financial or family pressures were too great."

"But there's only twenty-eight of you," I pointed out.

"Of course. That's because six of our original group aren't studying here in Sanare, but are still at medical school. They're studying in Cuba." With five of their initial group not continuing beyond their first or second year, the dropout rate was slightly more than 10 percent, well under the national rate of 26 percent reported by MIC nationwide analysis of the program.

Integration with the Community

The medical students in Monte Carmelo received encouragement from many friends and neighbors, including Elsy Perez, a practical nurse. She had been an original member of the village health committee when the first Cuban doctors arrived in 2004, and she continued to spend time volunteering at the *ambulatorio* even though she had a paid job at the small municipal hospital in nearby Sanare. On evenings and weekends, Elsy devoted her time to studying for a nursing degree in the Mission Sucre university program. One day, Elsy and a group of nursing and medical students were discussing the Venezuelan doctors they know, including the five employed at the Sanare municipal hospital. They felt that some of them, possibly because they were trained years ago in the established medical schools in the big cities, had a cold and distant manner with their patients. One nurse said there was a clear pattern of some patients being treated much better than others by the Venezuelan doctors at the hospital where she worked with Elsy. She attributed this to their class prejudices, for they seemed to assume that poor campesinos were stupid or incapable of understanding explanations of their maladies and treatment. This was in stark contrast to the Cuban doctors, she said. "They give everyone equal attention and treatment and put people at ease with their relaxed and friendly style. Everyone calls them by their first names."

There were, however, a couple of sympathetic Venezuelan general practitioners in Sanare who over the years had gained the trust of families in Monte Carmelo, and some older people kept going to them for treatment. One nursing student joked about her uncle, who received a free examination and antibiotics for bronchitis from a Cuban doctor at the Diagnostic Center in Sanare. Afterwards he went to the old family doctor and had the diagnosis confirmed. "I guess," she said, "he had some extra money that he needed to get rid of."

On another occasion, a first-year student from Monte Carmelo, Yeiny, told me that she too envisioned a different kind of medicine, one based on the same kind of humanitarian values that Arelys mentioned, but also connected to the folk medicine traditions of *el campo,* the countryside. As a child, Yeiny had developed a respect for the healing properties of native plants by watching local women, including her aunts, tend herb gardens with dozens of species that they used to treat such ailments as colds, flu, upset stomachs, and headaches. In the years when she had stopped attending school and was raising her infant son, she furthered this interest in naturalistic medicine by working with Father Mario, the local priest who occasionally showed up at the church to preach a sermon, but spent most of his time laboring alongside the campesinos at the cooperative farm. Yeiny helped Mario in the mini-laboratory he had created for producing healing tinctures, teas, and other rural remedies gathered from hundreds of local plants. When she entered the MIC program at age twenty-seven, she appreciated the fact that even though most of her medical training with the Cuban doctors was based on conventional Western science, alternative medicine based on traditional folk remedies was not dismissed as irrelevant.

Learning at the Side of Physician-Tutors

Most of my observing of MIC students as they worked alongside their Cuban tutors took place at two ambulatory clinics in the villages of Monte Carmelo and Palo Verde, as well as the new CDI, the diagnostic center, in the middle of Sanare. On my first visit to Palo Verde, Dr. Barbara and her Venezuelan colleague, Dr. Edita, simply invited me into their consulting office, placed me in a chair between their two desks, and invited me to spend the morning watching and listening to a steady parade of patients as they were sent in from the reception area. There were seven medical students present, and even those in their first year, including two who were only nineteen years old, were wearing the same white cotton jackets as the doctors. They carried themselves with a sense of dignity, seriousness, and attention to detail that was inculcated by the Cuban professor-tutors; their comportment told the rest of the world that they were already trusted medical assistants. The community members who came for treatment, some of whom were personally acquainted with the students, seemed perfectly comfortable with this arrangement and never seemed anxious about their privacy. Even the presence of this gringo in the room did not seem to phase anyone, either. Good health clearly involved the whole community.

There was a small private room to one side where the doctors and students could take patients for physical examinations. But first they took extensive histories from them, as well as accounts of their symptoms and physical condition. Dr. Barbara, as the physician in charge of instruction, was insistent that her students ask questions of her at regular intervals, both in terms of the kind of information she was gathering in the interview and the kinds of physical manifestations she was looking for in the physical exam.

Dr. Tomasa was the only family physician in Monte Carmelo in 2007–08, and at one point had to take an extended leave to travel home to Cuba and make arrangements for the care of her aging parents, who were quite ill. When I returned to Monte Carmelo in early 2009 for a brief visit and dropped by the *ambulatorio* to say hello, I was told by townspeople that she had ended a two-year rotation in Venezuela early so that she could return home and look after her parents personally, for their condition had continued to deteriorate. Although she was preoccupied with these issues during her time in Monte Carmelo, she took her job very seriously. Students told me that she was even more insistent than Dr. Barbara about getting them to ask questions during the course of their morning hours together. According to Antonio, one of the students from Sanare, "She is always demanding more questions because she says that kind of inquisitiveness is one of the keys to being successful doctors."

Dr. Tomasa's own curiosity led her to wonder about the large number of rural women who had chronic bronchitis and other lung and respiratory problems, yet they, unlike the men, seldom smoked cigarettes. At the time, she and the other Barrio Adentro physicians were eager to make maximum use of the laboratory and imaging capabilities of the Barrio Adentro II Diagnostic Center in Sanare in order to develop a coherent baseline of information on every resident, healthy or not. She decided to ask her medical students to try to set up appointments for as many Monte Carmelo residents as possible, but especially women, for chest X rays, blood counts, and other standard tests. If they were not comfortable going on their own, then the students could accompany them. The results of the X rays of women, even those who weren't coughing or ill, often showed shadowy congested areas in the lungs, just as if they had been heavy smokers. While the damp and cool weather during the rainy seasons probably contributed to these conditions, there was now evidence of another villain: the smoke from the wood fires that many women still used for cooking, often in closed rooms with low ceilings and no chimneys or other forms of proper ventilation.

This kind of intensive investigation of community health problems makes students aware at the beginning of their careers how important it is to analyze the particular environmental and social conditions of the locality in which they work, and then, through their familiarity and trust with the community, promote disease prevention. The students were effective in getting local residents to participate in vaccination campaigns, and they helped enlist and motivate schoolchildren during the rainy seasons in efforts to eliminate sources of standing water that serve as breeding areas for the little mosquitoes that spread dengue fever. And, since most medical students were young people who were generally putting off having children for a while, they were ideally suited to talking with their peers about sex and the various forms of birth control that were available.

New Compañeros *from Suriname*

Most residents of Monte Carmelo are descended in part from indigenous people who lived in the foothills of the Andes for thousands of years. Beginning in the sixteenth century, the Indians began intermarrying with European colonists who started coming inland from the coast to settle and with African slaves who rebelled on sugar plantations and escaped to live in the mountains. Distinct indigenous languages and tribal customs disappeared in this part of the country, and the traditional dances and music that are performed have had a mixture of Indian, Spanish, and African elements for hundreds of years. As for physical appearance, most people are brown-skinned with a range of facial features that testify to their mixed ethnic heritage.

One day in January of 2008, the residents of Monte Carmelo started whispering because three young people, apparently of Afro-Caribbean descent and wearing white jackets, were seen on the main road of Monte Carmelo with some other medical students. Were they from Barlovento, the people wondered, the part of Venezuela near the coast that is populated by the descendents of *cimarrones*, the rebellious slaves who centuries earlier escaped to the rain forests and built their own free towns? Or were they Afro-Cubans, like the popular Dr. Frank, the intensive-care physician at the diagnostic center in Sanare?

Later, when I was strolling past the *ambulatorio*, the students called me over to meet their three new *compañeros*. One of the newcomers, Georgo, identified me right away, "I think I detect an American accent in your Spanish." He was also speaking with an American accent, but in English. He said that Dutch was his native language because he came from Suriname, but English was an important language at the high school and university level in his country. Georgo, his half sister Isabella, and their friend Meredith were part of a contingent of foreign students that arrived in Venezuela in 2007 under the auspices of ELAM, the Latin American School of Medicine in Havana, in order to begin study alongside the MIC students. After completing premedical courses at a location outside of Caracas, these 335 doctors-in-training were dispersed into first-year classes with Venezuelan students at various locations all over the country. About half of the whole group came from Bolivia, others from Spanish American countries, and a fair number from non-Spanish-speaking cultures, such as Brazil and Suriname.

Georgo had been a top student in Paramaribo, the capital of Suriname, but had missed out when they held the lottery for places at the nation's tiny medical school. He started searching for other ways to study medicine, found that there was a long waiting period to become eligible for schools in the Netherlands, and that U.S. medical schools were prohibitively expensive. He first heard about Cuban medical training from Suriname's minister of health, who had studied medicine in Cuba himself, but found that there was an extremely long waiting list to get into the Latin American Medical School (ELAM). Dr. Juan Carrizo, rector of ELAM, has acknowledged that the number of applicants has grown so large that the school can only accept one out of twenty qualified students.

When Georgo learned that a special branch of ELAM was starting up in Venezuela, he and his sister Isabella applied directly through the Venezuelan embassy in Suriname for admission to the program. Karen, another new student from Peru, said that many of the forty Peruvians who arrived in Caracas had applied through socialist youth groups. Many of them, including Karen, had previously applied for admission to the Latin American School of Medicine in Havana, but had also been put on waiting lists. In the spring of 2008, as these students began their first year of regular medical studies with MIC, another contingent of 600 foreign students selected by ELAM arrived in Venezuela to begin the premedical course. (Georgo moved to Cuba the following year to study at the main ELAM campus. He reported that he liked the academic classes he was attending in Cuba, but that the practical experience he was getting in medical settings in Havana did not compare with the richness of his daily experience alongside the Cuban doctors and Venezuelan students in Barrio Adentro.)

Classes with First-Year Students

A week after meeting the new students, I was able to attend an afternoon class with the twenty first-year medical students, thirteen from the greater Sanare area plus the seven new foreign arrivals. Dr. Alina, who worked mornings at a Barrio Adentro consulting office in a poor neighborhood of Sanare, began her class with the thirteen students from the Sanare area by giving them a short quiz on molecular genetics, the previous week's focus of study. The other seven—three from Suriname, two from Colombia, one from Brazil, and one from Peru—waited patiently outside on the street because they had not been present for the first two weeks of classes.

After the quiz, Dr. Alina brought the foreign students into the group and asked everyone if they could explain some concepts related to the quiz. Arelys from Monte Carmelo had no problem concisely explaining the interactions among XX and XY and XYY chromosomes. Then the doctor turned to one of the foreign students who were in the process of catching up on the readings and asked him to set up a six-part chart related to "*operadores, promotores, regulatores, y cistrones.*" This particular student appeared a bit lost and had a sheepish grin on his face as he struggled to write things on the board. The grin did not appear to amuse the doctor, and though she refrained from scolding him, she did suggest to the whole group that in this class a serious commitment to study was necessary. She turned to another newcomer, Georgo, and repeated the same question, and he had no difficulty charting a diagram and explaining the required processes in detail.

Up until this point everyone had been squeezed into a crowded reception room that had a street door on one side, and in the opposite corner a desk and a computer for Dr. Humberto, who served as director of education activities at the MIC center. He and Dr. Frank from the diagnostic center were huddled around a computer, discussing cardiac-arterial blockages, searching the Internet for various research data, and jotting down extensive notes related to the problem they had to solve. When the third-year students finished their class in an adjoining classroom, the first-year students moved into this larger room, which was quieter and equipped with old-fashioned school desks, plus a computer and large television for showing DVD films.

Dr. Alina split the class time with the film. About 70 percent was devoted to the doctor's crisp lecturing and 30 percent to the film over a period of two and half hours. The film was a well-made combination of animation, charts, and diagrams accompanied by a succinct and informative explication by a female narrator. This was not what I expected, for I had developed the erroneous impression that films used in classes were made from traditional lectures presented by professors in Cuban universities. Perhaps this was because a pastiche of VHS tapes and old slide shows had been used briefly in 2006 when MIC instruction began but had now been replaced by a comprehensive set of DVDs. This collection, designed to encompass the entire MIC curriculum, presented the subject matter for each week and each module of the six-year program. Just as important for the transmission of this knowledge was that during the previous two years the Cuban physician-tutors had returned to classes themselves; having studied the educational concepts that underlie the MIC curriculum and style of the DVDs, they were prepared to weave the content of the films into their classroom presentations.

During the first class I attended, Dr. Alina started up a DVD that announced that we were watching "Human Morphophysiology: Part Two, 1st trimester, 1st year." Since the film was designed to be an interactive tool, Dr. Alina made frequent use of the remote to stop and start the action whenever she felt like it. She was sharp and animated as she added detail, emphasized related material, and repeated the information in a fresh way to make sure the students were comprehending things. She urged them to raise their hands and ask questions at any time.

The general theme, which followed naturally on the previous week's genetic material, was human reproduction: how the cells of a baby are formed and how a normal pregnancy is achieved. A title page announced associated themes: "Gametogenesis, Fertilization, Development of the Zygote, Alterations, Contraception." After the film presented the different patterns of chromosomal joining and specific exceptional cases, Dr. Alina pointed out some of the abnormal processes that were most likely to lead to birth defects. Later, after the film showed the way in which the fertilized egg is implanted on the wall of the womb, she spent considerable time answering questions from students about unsuccessful pregnancies and the kinds of incorrect implantation that can lead to spontaneous abortions, entopic pregnancies, and so on. "This is the kind of material you need to master," she said, "because some day you're going to have to explain these processes to some of your patients."

After the doctor delved into "*blastocistos, zona pelucida, trofoblasto*" and other exotic (for me, at least) definitions, there was considerable discussion of the "feminine sexual cycle." The doctor suggested that there were various ways to help women understand their individual variations from the average length of the period and the time of ovulation, including the use of a rectal thermometer. As it turned out, this discussion was related to the students' first homework assignment, a rather straightforward task: they were asked to describe in detail the processes of ovogenesis and spermatogenesis.

A little later, Dr. Alina had a different kind of homework question. She asked the students to consider the hypothetical case of a truck driver who is on the road most of the month and is married to a woman who travels throughout the country regularly to promote one of the new social missions in Venezuela. They've been married for three years and she can't get pregnant. "What would you, as their doctor," she asked, "advise them to discuss? And what simple measures could they take to better their chances of having a child?"

A student from Colombia waved his hand and said, "I think I read an article about long-distance truckers and the possibility that because of all the time they spend sitting immobile in the cab this is cutting down on their sperm production."

The doctor rolled her eyes toward the ceiling, and then shook her head emphatically, "No, no, no, that's a bit of hypothetical speculation that comes out of the popular press. While it may or may not be true, there is a more straightforward approach that should probably solve this couple's problem, and you should try that first."

Her last homework question was intended to introduce them, as young medical people, to one of their roles as practitioners of comprehensive community medicine. As communicators responsible for improving public awareness of various health issues, they would have to share their knowledge with others and develop sympathy for the people they are treating. "You are in your Barrio Adentro office in a poor barrio, and a young girl comes in and says, 'I think I'm pregnant. But I don't know how I got pregnant.' What do you need to ask her? What do you need to explain to her?"

At another class a few weeks later, Dr. Alina paced the aisles between the students, pulling a full-sized replica of a human skeleton behind her on a little cart. The lesson began with students being quizzed on the spinal column and the functions of the different kinds of vertebrae. The three students from Suriname, always ready to answer, had their hands in the air. "You're too eager," said Dr. Alina, "keep your hands down." The other students, especially the local campesinos, laughed because they were amused by the sibling rivalry between Georgo and his sister, Isabella. Or perhaps they might have been reacting to urban students, raised in the capital of Suriname (not exactly a huge metropolitan center, with about 250,000 people, but ten times the size of the town of Sanare) who had a more competitive style since they had been sent to high-powered schools with instruction in both Dutch and English.

"Let's hear from some other students," said the doctor. "Yeiny? Please give us three features of the thoracic vertebrae." Yeiny, a twenty-eight-year-old student from Monte Carmelo, gave a correct and comprehensive answer in her soft voice.

Another question: "Why are the lumbar vertebrae larger?" Isabella's hand shot up so quickly that Dr. Alina teased her. "You're sure to strain a muscle in your arm if you don't stop." Then the doctor ignored her and called on José, the oldest member of the class.

"They're bigger," he said, "because they're at the bottom of the whole spinal column and have to support more weight." Then he successfully answered some other detailed questions about spinal functions.

For the next hour, Dr. Alina, accompanied by her skeleton, asked the students questions, invited them to ask her questions, and described hypothetical dilemmas of diagnosis that might confront a local doctor. "There is a guy who drank too many beers and he takes off on his motorcycle on a country road"—a fairly common occurrence in the surrounding area—"and he can't negotiate the curve and tumbles across the road. He doesn't seem to have broken any arms and legs, or his skull, but he's having trouble breathing and his lungs are filling up with fluid. One possibility," she explained and pointed to her skeleton companion, "is that one of these, a floating rib, has punctured his lung."

Next the DVD reviewed the *"sistema osteomioarticular,"* the skeletal system. It began with a look at a baby's embryo in the third week, the first location of bone cells in the sixth week, the beginning of large bone formation in the eighth week, first the arms, then the legs two days later. At one point Dr. Alina stopped the film to speak briefly about minor birth defects in the skeletal system that may be due to inherited characteristics, such as missing or extra fingers and toes, then said, 'We'll study much more about various kinds of birth defects and their potential causes, both genetic and environmental, when you get to your third year."

When homework assignments were given, the first question was: "I want you to describe all the differences in bone structures and connective tissue between males and females, giving particular attention to everything below the waist, including pelvis, legs, and hips." And then Dr. Alina pointed out that she wanted the normal differences:

"For example, one thing you would expect to find would be greater density in men's bones compared to women's. What was startling to us as we examined men and women in Venezuela over the past several years, especially in poor rural areas and barrios where we Barrio Adentro doctors are working, is that there is not necessarily much difference in the bone density of adult men and women. This can be due to only one thing—the inadequate diet that many Venezuelans have had over most of their lifetimes."

The second homework assignment suggested a role that these students might be playing in the future if they were to serve in the rain forest in an isolated part of Venezuela or Brazil. "You are a doctor serving an indigenous community in the state of Amazonas. A young child is found wandering about, and none of the local people know who he is. He appears to be very small, but then most of the people in this area are short in stature. You, the doctor, are asked to determine how old he is, and since you have an x-ray machine at your disposal, you do a film of his hand. You see that part of the hand is not totally ossified, that is, the bones are not totally formed. Tell me some characteristics of these bones that you would look for so you could indicate his approximate age."

Mission Sucre: El Plan Extraordinario

Although many of the components of the Medicina Integral Comunitaria curriculum migrated to Venezuela with the Cubans, MIC was able to be implemented in hundreds of Venezuelan municipalities at once because the nation had launched an alternative Bolivarian education system. Under the various education missions that began functioning after the year 2000, millions of Venezuelans had the opportunity to complete their elementary and secondary education or advance to some form of higher university or technical training.

Mission Robinson began by teaching the illiterate to read and write, and then it quickly evolved into Mission Robinson II, which guided students through six grades of primary school material. Mission Ribas allowed others to complete their high school studies, and many of these, both young and older adults, wanted to continue studying at the university level courses. These people, along with those who had once completed conventional high school but never had the opportunity to attend traditional universities, were admitted by the hundreds of thousands into El Plan Extraordinario Mariscal Antonio José de Sucre, or Mission Sucre. A variety of fields were open to them; some of the most popular are social science, computer science, agro-ecology, law, nursing, sports training, scientific technology, and education.

At the end of 2010, there were more than two million university-level students in Venezuela, about three times as many as when Chávez assumed the presidency. Most of them were studying in institutions that did not exist eight years earlier. Approximate numbers suggest that about 400,000 students were studying at the conventional public institutions, including various teachers' colleges and technical colleges, and the elite schools like Central University of Venezuela in Caracas; about 600,000 were studying at the private universities and colleges, many of them connected to the Catholic Church; about 500,000 studied at the new Bolivarian and the expanded experimental universities; and about 600,000 were enrolled in the *universidad extra muros,* or "university without walls," that is found all over the country in the form of Mission Sucre; it was serving the same number of students, 600,000, as were enrolled in the entire traditional system of higher education when President Chávez was first elected in 1998.

By 2008, graduates of Mission Sucre programs in primary and secondary education were teaching in Bolivarian schools. Jesús, who did his student teaching in Monte Carmelo, was hired to teach in a *liceo* in Sanare. A young graduate who lived next door to us in Monte Carmelo traveled five hours by jeep into the forests of the Yacambú valley every Sunday evening. She lived there with a family during the week and taught young children of various ages in a one-room school house, then rode home by jeep on Friday evenings.

Each municipality in Venezuela (equivalent to a county in the United States) has a Mission Sucre central office and coordinators who enroll students for the various programs. Though it helps recruit and interview students for the MIC medical program, Mission Sucre's main duty is providing other university educational programs in local communities. Many of these—such as nursing, sports training, physical rehabilitation, and medical technology—play obvious supporting roles in ensuring community health and well-being.

There are other ways that Mission Sucre contributes to community-wide consciousness of public health. For instance, every student who is matriculating in social science has to work as part of a team that identifies a problem or concern of a local community. Aside from their conventional course work, the student's team has to build their final thesis around a problem identified in meetings with this community, then researches the social science literature for analysis of this particular problem, and concludes with written and audiovisual material that suggests possible solutions for the community. In order to graduate, students must take part in a public forum where they present their findings to interested citizens from all over the municipality and, in particular, to the small community or neighborhood that was the focus of their study.

Often these thesis projects have direct relation to community health problems that can be solved or ameliorated. Social science student Carmen Alicia, a grandmother from Monte Carmelo (and mother of Yeiny, the first-year medical student), worked with two young women from the neighboring village of Bojó on the long-term problem of eliminating the threats posed by pesticides for local campesinos and their families. Although the community had already cut its pesticide use by 60 percent and some individuals and cooperatives were engaged in organic farming, they could show that it was still of great importance to wean farmers away from poisonous chemicals and introduce them to healthier methods of farming. One of the major objectives was to eliminate pesticides in human breast milk. To convince their neighbors that this was important, the students gathered evidence from medical studies in the state of Lara. In the nearby city of Quibor, 80 percent of nursing mothers had their milk contaminated by agricultural pesticides. In an investigation of 15,000 births at the hospital in Barquisimeto in 1990, the rate of birth defects was five times higher than the national average. A similar study in 2004 showed that this rate had increased to eleven times greater than the average.

Elsy, the health committee volunteer, was also working on a Mission Sucre thesis in her nursing program. Only one person from Monte Carmelo had ever completed a university nursing degree in the past, and she had managed this by living with relatives in the city of

Barquisimeto. Elsy and forty-six other students were completing a three-year course to become licensed nurses; if they completed another two-year program they could earn the equivalent of a Bachelor of Science degree in nursing. For their final thesis project, she and three classmates evaluated the current health needs of the village of Monte Carmelo. Among other recommendations, they identified the need for better public recreation facilities and advised improvements to the only small sports area that existed in the village, an asphalt basketball court that was also used for volleyball and *futbolito* (a small-scale soccer game). They suggested constructing a *concha*, or open-air roof, since rain limited the use of the area during the wet seasons, and hot sun kept the children off the area during midday in other months of the year. After Elsy's group made a public presentation of their findings, they took their proposal to the village community council and requested federal money to fund the construction.

Missions: Dedication to Education

In June 2005, when I made my first visit to the Sanare-Monte Carmelo area, I was fortunate to meet Honorio Dam, the director of rural teachers for the municipality of Andres Eloy Blanco. Over the years, Honorio had worked with a remarkable corps of teachers who were willing to devote themselves to experimental schools and the daunting task of serving the people in 123 hamlets and thousands of little farms scattered through the deeply creased landscape of steep mountains and precipitous valleys. Many of the teachers were progressive Catholics who had been influenced by the educational philosophy of Paolo Freire and liberation theology, and who, long before Chávez came to power, had initiated experimental programs that benefited campesinos. They were unanimous in their support of the Chávez government not only because it materially improved the lives of the poor and marginalized, but also because the education missions and construction of new rural high schools opened up the possibility of revolutionizing educational practice.

"The biggest change in Venezuela," Honorio insisted, "is that millions of Venezuelans are in school in 2005 who were not being educated in 1997." By 2009, the statistics were definitely bearing him out: 437,000 adults had graduated from Mission Robinson elementary education; 510,000 from Mission Ribas secondary education; and over 600,000 had enrolled in Mission Sucre or already graduated. Free day care was available to three- to five-year-old children with 66 percent attending; elementary school attendance had risen from 86 percent to 93 percent, and many of these schools now offered students two free meals a day; attendance at the high school level was up, from 47 to 68 percent, and the number of students in higher education had more than doubled thanks to the creation of new Bolivarian universities and the Mission Sucre program.

Honorio Dam invited me to accompany him to the first Mission Ribas graduation ceremony in Sanare in June of 2005, a major event in which fifty-eight people, mostly women, were honored by local dignitaries including the mayor. Many of the rural teachers offered eloquent testimony on behalf of the graduating students; often they had known them as children and then taught them again, years later, as adults. As they recounted the hardships these students had overcome in order to complete their high school degrees, the teachers did not call attention to their own sacrifices; they had given up their free time in the evenings and on weekends to serve as volunteer teachers in the first Mission Ribas classes. The friends, families, and in many cases, the children of the graduates were attending the ceremony, giving it a very festive atmosphere.

When the ceremonies were concluded, many of the graduates were talking excitedly about their future university education and the courses of study they wanted to pursue. When I reviewed my notes from this 2005 trip five years later, I noticed one that referred to a mayor on TV who suggested that five of the outstanding graduates from Mission Ribas in his municipality were going to travel to Cuba to study medicine the following year. My notation reads: "!!??
Que cosa es ??!!"—What's this??!! I suppose I thought the mayor had been engaging in political hyperbole, for at the time I wasn't

aware that Venezualan campesinos were already going to ELAM for medical school.

I also was unaware of developments that were more unbelievable. That summer, over 24,000 students all over Venezuela were enrolling in the MIC premedical qualifying course. By the following January, those who performed well in the course would begin the first year of a six-year medical education. Undoubtedly some of the women I had seen at the Mission Ribas ceremony were definitely going to medical school—if not in Cuba, then certainly at home in their own community.

9. Revolutionary Medicine in Conflict with the Past

Is it an inevitable fact, that universities should become conservative or even flashpoints for reaction?

—CHE GUEVARA, 1959

"During the three years that a doctor remains here doing a postgraduate residency, he earns a salary that doesn't permit him to live independently, to have his own house or vehicle, or raise a family." This is how José, a traditional medical student enrolled at Universidad Central de Venezuela in Caracas, Venezuela's most prestigious public university, explained why he was choosing to go to Spain in 2009 to do his residency training.[1]

Arelys, a young mother and nontraditional medical student enrolled in Medicina Integral Comunitaria in Sanare, state of Lara, explained why she was looking forward to a future of working as a community physician within the Barrio Adentro system: "We are thinking of medicine as a vocation, our calling in life, our way of serving the people and building socialist values. We don't want a profession in the old sense, where many doctors were motivated by a desire for money and prestige, and wanted to feel that they were superior to the patients, the nurses, and everyone else."[2]

In 2009, José was quoted in a major Caracas newspaper that, like the vast majority of the private media in Venezuela, has been opposed to President Chávez ever since he took office in 1999. The article implied that the country's medical system was on the verge of collapse because José and some other students, an estimated 20 percent of medical graduates from traditional universities, were applying for residencies abroad, especially in Spain. There was no mention of any nontraditional medical students like Arelys who are studying Medicina Integral Comunitaria; the extraordinary increase in teh number of MIC students was generally ignored by the private media, even though by 2009 they vastly outnumbered the traditional university medical students.

José has not been quoted here in order to belittle him, for his kind of thinking is probably typical of most young doctors around the world, who believe they should be well rewarded for the practice of their profession. Nor is the phenomenon of brain drain new or unique, for an estimated 10 percent of young Venezuelan doctors were leaving for Spain and other countries before Hugo Chávez became president. In the poorest developing countries of the world, much higher percentages of medical graduates, often over 50 percent, are accustomed to leave for the greener pastures of the cities and suburbs in the rich industrialized countries. But one reason that the rate of desertion may be increasing in Venezuela is that there is conflict between two different medical systems, the traditional capitalist-oriented model favoring private services for the wealthy and middle classes, and the new Bolivarian model dispensing universal public care through Barrio Adentro. Clearly this is not just a medical conflict, but also a class conflict of the kind that Che Guevara encountered in Cuba fifty years earlier.

In October of 1959, only ten months after the victorious guerrilla army had entered Havana, Che visited university campuses and found that many students were less than enthusiastic about transforming their society. These students, according to Che's biographer Paco

Ignacio Taibo II, were "on the sidelines, and in keeping with their professors' liberal opposition to the government, were resisting pressure to join the revolutionary process."[3] The Argentinian Che entered into a lively debate with students at the University of Oriente Province in Santiago de Cuba and challenged their ideas. "Is it an inevitable fact," he asked them, "that universities should become conservative or even flashpoints for reaction?"

Che was not speaking to future doctors, since the city of Santiago de Cuba did not yet have a medical school. But he was hoping he could win over some of these young people to the side of the revolution despite the fact that most of them came from middle- and upper-class families that did not have revolutionary aspirations for their children. The students had been sent to university with the expectation that they would manage businesses or practice well-rewarded professions. Very soon they would not have those choices. By 1960 and 1961, the direction of the revolution was determined, and privileged young people were asked to adapt to the egalitarian expectations of the new Cuba. Although some of them would decline the invitation and end up abandoning their country, it remains remarkable that so many university students actually did go forth to serve impoverished campesinos, either by working in the literacy campaigns or with the Rural Medical Service, and later became the backbone of new and completely different health and education systems. Though they were no doubt energized by youthful idealism, they also were the beneficiaries of the one precondition that, according to Che's 1960 speech "On Revolutionary Medicine," was necessary to overturn the old medical and social order: "For one to be a revolutionary doctor or to be a revolutionary at all, there must first be a revolution."

Bolivarian Revolution: A Different Course

The Bolivarian Revolution has followed a much different course than the Cuban Revolution. In Venezuela, there was no military victory that signaled the arrival of the revolution and the defeat of the old ruling powers. The Bolivarian process has followed a deliberate path of reform and peaceful organization within the existing capitalist society, with the intention of ultimately achieving a new form of democratic socialism. It was not until President Chávez had been in office for five years that he first spoke explicitly about socialism to a group of international writers and artists, presenting a very heterodox version, in which the teachings of Jesus and the activities of Bolivar were as prominent as the analysis of Marx.[4] A few months later, at the World Social Forum held in Brazil in early 2005, he shared his expansive political vision with the larger world and called it "Socialism for the 21st Century." From that point on his message has been unique, yet fairly consistent at its core; in 2010 Chávez was still concluding his weekly opinion column, "Las Lineas de Chávez," with the words, "Con Marx, con Cristo, con Bolívar." The Bolivarian Revolution, with its new strands of socialist thought and practice, has been developing over more than a decade, and at the same time the Venezuelan capitalist class has continued to maintain most of its property and material advantages. A large portion of the upper-middle class has been trying to protect its old privileges of cultural and educational dominance, including access to the best professional careers. These privileged minorities exercise a strong reactionary force in opposition to the progressive tide of the revolution. Many, perhaps most, students at the traditional public and private universities in Venezuela believe they deserve the advantages inherited from their parents, and they are also immersed in the U.S-dominated global consumer culture that keeps them focused on expectations of high material rewards. It is not surprising, now that they are living in a more equitable society, that they are afraid career paths that once led to high earnings and social prestige, such as the practice of medicine, will be blocked.

The Chávez administration, however, has not interfered very much with the old models of providing private medical care or the training of medical doctors at the traditional universities. Health care for less than 20 percent of the population continues to be funded by private insurance companies and delivered by specialists who work in private clinics and were trained, just like José, at the nation's best universities. The cost of this kind of care, which was too expensive for 80 percent of the population when Chávez was first elected in 1998, was still prohibitively expensive in 2010. Likewise, the Chávez government has not interfered with other kinds of private business; for example, the developers of fancy shopping malls and gated housing communities—the late twentieth-century emblems of private property rights—kept building like crazy when the economy was booming from late 2003 through 2008. In general, business in the private sector and private spending by all citizens was not curtailed by President Chávez or by state and local governments. Instead, the federal government spent most of its energy and revenues on developing a parallel world of social missions that have enhanced the quality of life for the large majority of the population and now serve as the basis for building alternative, nationwide institutions, such as a system of universal, free public health care.

"El divorcio de la clase media alta"
The Divorce of the Upper Middle Class

In the spring of 2009, I spoke with Cuban writer and philosopher Enrique Ubieta Gómez about the ten months he spent touring Venezuela in 2005 and 2006. He had visited Barrio Adentro locations in all twenty-four Venezuelan states and interviewed hundreds of people—Cuban doctors in Barrio Adentro, barrio residents, campesinos, millionaires, private newspaper editors, medical entrepreneurs in plastic surgery, and promoters of beauty contests. He then published *Venezuela rebelde: solidaridad versus dinero*[5] (Rebel Venezuela: Solidarity vs. Money), which not only records the experiences of contemporary Venezuela as well as any recent book, but also highlights the major battle that is being waged, a struggle between a democratic majority relying on new commitments of social solidarity and an entrenched but fading minority trying to maintain its power through the capital it controls.

The enormous separation between rich and poor is not a matter of incomes diverging, since careful economic analysis by organizations such as the Center for Economic and Policy Research in Washington has demonstrated that the poorest 80 percent of the population have been steadily gaining a larger share of the national income. The Gini coefficient, the standard measure of inequality, has been diminishing significantly, and by 2009, Venezuela, one of the richest countries per capita in South America, became the nation with the most equal income distribution. Ubieta believes that even though the upper strata of society might be losing ground in economic statistics, the great divide between the classes was widening—for political and cultural reasons. This was the result of *"el divorcio de la clase media alta"*— the divorce of the upper-middle class—a separation from the rest of Venezuelan society that was becoming permanent.

The "divorce" probably began with the desire of the upper classes to increasingly isolate themselves from other Venezuelans as their society was deteriorating in the 1980s and 1990s. As in most Latin American countries, much of the growing inequality and social misery was engendered by neoliberal privatization, obsequious acceptance of the rule of global finance, and cutbacks in public services. At the same time, the increasing globalization of consumer culture was being accelerated by television, the Internet, and by the experiences of upper-class tourists and students, who saw Miami and the United States as worthy of emulation. In the long run, however, this divorce wasn't one-sided, because after the privileged began the process, Chávez was elected and the popular classes decided they did not need to pander to the whims of a spoiled, demanding, and paternalistic upper-middle class any longer.

With the advent of Barrio Adentro and other participatory activities, the lower classes took such an active role in the political life of the country that they did not automatically respect the pronouncements of the opinion makers favored by the rich. The Chávez government made sure that cultural venues that were once attended mostly by upper-class audiences, such as the Teresa Carreño National Theatre in downtown Caracas, encouraged the attendence of all people, including those from the lower classes. On one occasion when I was in Caracas, the thousands of seats in the auditorium were packed with enthusiastic citizens who had been admitted free to an international poetry festival. I was told by a friend that many rich Caracans had stopped attending such cultural events, even the orchestral musical performances, complaining that "it smells in there." Apparently, as far as they were concerned, the theater had been contaminated by the great unwashed.

Because the Chávez administration allied itself in solidarity with the majority of the people, the divorced upper-middle class became more and more marginalized. In the economic sense, most suffered very little, but in the sense of social prestige and social power, they were more and more frustrated by their inability to control the increasingly more democratic apparatus of the state and by their diminishing esteem in the eyes of the general public. It was as if the rest of the population had told them: "We are going to create our own social reality built on our own values."

The process of increasingly severe class stratification that began in the 1980s was exacerbated in the 1990s and affected Venezuela the same way it had most nations: neoliberal policies were starving public services while cutting taxes for the rich. In this atmosphere, new entrance exams for the elite public universities were introduced that favored upper-class students educated in private schools and excluded more and more lower-class students. During a discussion that local school teachers were having with sociologist Carlos Ganz in a rural part of Lara in March of 2008, one participant cited statistics concerning the students at UCV (Central University of Venezuala in Caracas, the most prestigious public university in the country). Two and three decades earlier, he said, nearly 20 percent of UCV students came from the "*clases populares*" (meaning poor and working classes); but after the year 2000 only 4 percent did.[6] One reason for this was that as less money was appropriated for public education by the state in the 1980s and 1990s, more and more upper- and middle-class students were attending private secondary schools that could afford to give them better preparation for the competitive entrance exams for the university.

Just as public education was starved for government funds, so was public health care, with the result that primary care and hospital care in public facilities deteriorated rapidly. This coincided with the pre-ponderance of middle- and upper-class students obtaining profes-sional degrees at the universities, who were predisposed to look for opportunites in lucrative private medical clinics rather than enter public service. On the other hand, not all Venezuelan graduates of the traditional medical schools sought to make a lot of money in private practice, either because of a desire to work with the underserved majority or simply because the private sector was limited and could only absorb a finite number of physicians to work with 20 percent of the population. Long before Chávez came to power, thousands of doc-tors worked in public hospital jobs that were not well compensated. Many of them were frustrated by the poor condition of hospital facili-ties, the failure to integrate their workplaces with the Barrio Adentro system, and the delays in raising pay that persisted during the early years of the Chávez government, even after increasing oil revenues that were sufficient for improving the situation. For example, it was not until 2010 that salary levels and extra benefits were increased and equalized for physicians working in two different kinds of public facil-ities, the Ministry of Health hospitals and the social security hospitals (which had enjoyed a system of meaningful bonus payments for many years). This was not necessarily prejudicial treatment of dentists, doc-tors, and nurses working within the old public system, because even those who worked in Barrio Adentro had to campaign to achieve deserved raises. The approximately 2,500 Venezuelan doctors who had trained at the traditional universities and then took the step of completing residencies in comprehensive community medicine made conscious decisions to support the Bolivarian process and work as colleagues of the Cuban doctors in Barrio Adentro I and II. Some of these physicians took the lead in exposing the shortcomings of the national health ministry.

Dr. Adolfo Delgado, president of the Bolivarian Society of General Comprehensive Medicine, the organization representing Venezuelans who work in various medical capacities within Barrio Adentro, pub-lished a series of letters in the pages of *Aporrea*, a busy online site fea-turing news, opinion, and energetic muckraking. He pushed for wage increases that had been promised to Barrio Adentro doctors in 2008 and led a spirited fight that succeeded in ousting national Minister of Health Jesus Mantilla in 2009, who was blamed by many for permitting some Barrio Adentro programs to deteriorate. In one public protest attended by many of his colleagues, Delgado proposed drastic changes in the national coordination of Barrio Adentro: "Regional committees of the Barrio Adentro Foundation should be either eliminated or reorganized; in 90 percent of cases they have been ineffective in responding to the problems of staffing, equipment and pay."

During these protests, Dr. Delgado had to make it clear that he and other revolutionary doctors in the organization had no interest in paralyzing the public health service. This was because the political opposition had been propagandizing against Barrio Adentro ever since it was instituted, and was urging public physicians to sabotage the new health system. Delgado estimated that about 10 percent of the public doctors might be influenced by campaigns that were urging them to go on strike, and declared, "We will not fall for this game of the opposition, who want us to abandon our posts of duty." In March 2009, a letter to *Aporrea* from Delgado and other doctors explained to readers that the delivery of primary care was the foundation of a new universal medical system, and that the Bolivarian constitution gave "priority to health promotion and disease prevention."[7] He warned that inattention to the complexities of expanding Barrio Adentro to levels II, III, and IV was endangering comprehensive community health services at their most important level, Barrio Adentro I.

This kind of active and accurate criticism by Dr. Delgado and many others had an effect, for the government appointed a new health minister who initiated a review of the shortcomings of Barrio Adentro. Later that summer, in August of 2009, President Chávez told a nationwide television audience that as many as 2,000 primary care sites of Barrio Adentro I were not functioning properly or were closed down entirely for lack of personnel. In the second address to the nation in October, he outlined the kinds of remedies that were being taken to restore proper service to the public, including the arrival of 1,000 more Cuban doctors before the end of the year. By

January of 2010, all of the Barrio Adentro I consulting offices were operational again.

The Political Opposition's Attacks on Barrio Adentro

Dr. Douglas Leon Natera, the head of the Venezuelan Medical Federation (the equivalent of the AMA), has been raising the alarm about Barrio Adentro ever since the first Cuban doctors arrived in 2003. For years he completely disparaged their activities, saying: "They gave them jobs without even seeing if they were doctors. This is causing big public health problems," and "We're being invaded by so-called doctors trained in Marxist-Leninism and the Castro-communism of the dictator of the Caribbean island of Cuba."[8] At that time, before the Chávez government had consolidated the Bolivarian process, extreme right-wingers felt they could intimidate the poor with violent verbal attacks; supporters of Coordinadora Democrática, the opposition group that led anti-Chávez rallies in 2003–4, waved signs that said, "Be a patriot, kill a Cuban doctor."[9] The following year, Oswaldo Alvarez Paz, the political director of another opposition group, claimed that "in the whole national territory more than 45 thousand Cubans with military training can be found, camouflaged in special activities such as doctors and paramedics, teachers, professors and sports trainers."[10] In 2008, ORVEX, the Organization of Venezuelans in Exile, which was funded by rich expatriates in Miami, managed to issue the most outrageous reaction when it released a short film titled *La Universidad del Terrorismo Patrocinada por del Gobierno de Venezuela*. According to this piece of disinformation that appeared on YouTube, "a university of terrorism" had been created at the Latin American School of Medicine (ELAM) in Havana, where terrorist doctors were being prepared to attack the entire Western Hemisphere under the patronage of Hugo Chávez and the Venezuelan government.

These verbal assaults on Barrio Adentro and Cuban medical training were accompanied by the refusal of some cities and states, still under the control of the political opposition, to allow the deployment of Barrio Adentro physicians. In 2003 in the city of Barcelona, capital of the state of Anzoátegui, Cuban doctor German Carreras arrived in a barrio that didn't have an empty space for a Barrio Adentro consulting office. The neighborhood health committee and medical personnel started rebuilding a dilapidated and abandoned police station to serve as temporary quarters for the medical mission. At the time, local government was under the control of a governor and mayor opposed to Chávez, and they decided to send law officers in to close down the makeshift clinic. They did not succeed, because 100 people showed up to surround the new office and block the police. The group swelled to 300 residents determined to defend their right to health care. The doctors kept working and the residents told the police, "If you want to pass through to remove the doctors, you have to do it over our dead bodies."[11] The police never bothered the Barrio Adentro office again. In 2004, voters in the state of Anzoátegui elected a pro-Chávez governor, the poet-lawyer Tarek William Saab, and since then Barrio Adentro facilities have been protected rather than threatened.

After 2004, opposition media and political forces had little success in attacking Barrio Adentro. Although many private medical practitioners remained antagonistic, there were also a significant number of well-established physicians who, because of their expertise and interest, were incorporated into Barrio Adentro and its supporting institutions. One of these was Dr. Claudio Letelier, the director of the first Barrio Adentro II hospital and diagnostic clinic that opened in Venezuela in 2004 and was located in the barrio of Caricuao outside of Caracas. Like most of the senior medical professionals who were in charge of the new Bolivarian health system, he was a product of the elite university system, but he nevertheless recognized the necessity of creating a new public health system. He also came from an elite family background. "I live in the eastern part of the city," Dr. Letelier told a reporter in 2005. "My family has an ultra-right background. We are a family of landowners. My parents did, however, also teach me about social responsibility. The health programs of this government are very beneficial for the people of Venezuela. I want to support them. That is why I am supporting this process. . . . Before, in some hospitals the situation was appalling. Patients were dying in the hallways because of a lack of doctors or medicine. Nowadays, most of the hospital directors are supporting the Bolivarian process."

Dr. Letelier's Barrio Adentro II hospital, which was staffed by Venezuelan personnel, had developed a very successful relationship with all seventy-two small ambulatory clinics in the barrio that were referring their patients. These clinics were all staffed by Cuban experts in comprehensive community medicine. "Unfortunately, some of the medical organizations in Venezuela are very politicized," said Dr. Letelier, "and claimed that all the Cuban doctors are communists and the quality of their work cannot be not as good as ours. The Cubans, however, come here to help. They are too professional to be occupied with politics; they come here on a purely humanitarian mission."[12]

Three or four years later, there were virtually no opposition spokespeople or aspirants for public office who were willing to say they wanted to shut down Barrio Adentro. This did not mean that attacks on Barrio Adentro ended. Because the representative political system in Venezuela remained democratic and open to competitive challenges from the right, a number of anti-Chávez candidates had been elected as mayors and governors in the fall of 2008, especially in areas where pro-Chávez incumbents were viewed to be incompetent or corrupt. A few angry supporters of the newly elected opposition felt their electoral success gave them license to renew open class warfare against the poor and began intimidating Barrio Adentro workers. For instance, employees of the Barrio Adentro II Integral Diagnostic Center in Los Dos Caminos neighborhood of the Sucre municipality in Caracas reported that members of Primera Justicia were threatening to burn down their medical building and were circulating a petition to remove the Cuban doctors. In the state of Carabobo, another place that had just elected an opposition governor, two Cuban doctors were gravely wounded when three men broke into their diagnostic center, destroyed valuable equipment, and attacked them.[13]

These limited mobilizations of violent antipathy gained no traction and were roundly condemned. The same was true of semi-legal tactics utilized to disrupt Barrio Adentro in the state of Miranda, where Henrique Capriles Radonsky, a vociferous right-wing Chávez opponent, was elected governor in 2008. In early 2009 the governor's office sent police to demand that twenty-five Cuban doctors vacate the premises of a large house that had been put at their disposal as living quarters in El Hatillo, a rich suburban area built around a quaint colonial town. Since the area is also home to a large minority of lower-income residents, Barrio Adentro had been serving both poor and mixed income neighborhoods. Neighbors of the Barrio Adentro facilities were not about to have their health care jeopardized, so they immediately mobilized seventy different community councils and surrounded the building with hundreds of supporters of the medical staff. They declared that they would not permit the local police or anyone else to evict their doctors. When the police and governor finally had no choice but to back down, a local lawyer, Omaira Camacho, made a point of informing reporters that it would be difficult to close down the Barrio Adentro facilities because they were not just serving the poor: "Many upper-middle-class residents of La Lagunita, La Boyera, and Los Naranjos," she said, "have been getting free consultations and treatment."[14]

In 2009, the government had not been maintaining parts of Barrio Adentro properly, and President Chávez had to publicly acknowledge the problem in detailed television addresses and then act swiftly to correct the shortcomings. The opposition and Dr. Leon Natera, head of the national medical association, were delighted with this setback, and once again used the anti-Chávez media to attack the president. But this time, rather than attack Barrio Adentro, he defended it. Whereas his claim that 80 percent of the Barrio Adentro consulting offices were not functioning was vastly exaggerated, his argument was bound to gain some traction with the public; he said that the Chávez government was so inefficient and corrupt that it was betraying the people of Venezuela by not operating Barrio Adentro properly.

A year later, in 2010, when all the seats in the Venezuelan National Assembly were due to be contested, Dr. Leon Natera of the medical association decided to run as an opposition candidate for the National

Assembly in March of 2010 in El Hatillo, the very community where officials had tried to remove the Cuban doctors the year before. He pledged that "we will verify that all the modules [the recently constructed Barrio Adentro consulting offices] that are closed will be opened again." (In reality, all of those offices had been restaffed and reopened by then, but obviously Leon Natera was not going to dispense with a good campaign promise.)

Some Shortcomings of Barrio Adentro

Although provocative attacks invented by the old medical establishment, repeated regularly in the private media, will not disappear as long as upper-class antagonism tries to undermine the Bolivarian Revolution, there remained problems with the development of Barrio Adentro that cannot be blamed on the opposition and were internal to the Bolivarian political and social process. Even though the program has been a stunning achievement because it has brought comprehensive health care within reach of almost all Venezuelans, it was pieced together so rapidly that some portions became difficult to manage. The rapid resuscitation of the understaffed Barrio Adentro consulting offices at the end of 2009 was possible because of the grassroots strength of local health committees and the sustained solidarity of Cuban medical personnel, who were able to supply a new infusion of volunteers. To date, there is no complete analysis of why Barrio Adentro experienced this shaky period, but a number of factors have been discussed over the past few years.[15]

1. Although Barrio Adentro primary care facilities were fully staffed within the first year of the program, 2003–04, most consulting offices were temporary affairs and not necessarily placed in the neighborhoods that would need them the most. In heavily populated city barrios, where residents numbered in the hundreds of thousands, some small neighborhoods had better coverage than others; some of the less organized communities had trouble maintaining the kind of health committee strength that was necessary to

generate the neighborhood support needed by Cuban and Venezuelan medical personnel.

2. Many Cuban doctors took on the formidable double duty of providing primary medical consultations in the mornings, and then preparing and teaching formal medical classes in the afternoons. At a great many locations, this meant that patients were no longer seen in the afternoons. There were also other disruptions, for many Cuban doctors who taught classes to Venezuelan students had to return to Cuba for short-term intensive courses and accreditation that would prepare them to deal with the new medical curriculum and computer-generated material.

3. Over time, the needs of the communities and the nature of patient visits changed. While in the first years of service, Cuban doctors regularly went house to house to gain the confidence of residents, this was not so necessary once people were comfortable going directly to the ambulatory clinics or the diagnostic centers. Some patients seemed to prefer the larger diagnostic centers because they were open for longer periods during the day and had more sophisticated facilities.

4. In any given locality, the schedules of doctors might be juggled due to the rotation of medical volunteers or other special situations. For example, when Dr. Tomasa returned to Cuba to care for her ailing parents (see chapter 8), another Cuban doctor had to divide his time with another community and be driven to Monte Carmelo to see patients two or three times a week.

5. In many areas, the need to respond to emergency and long-neglected health issues diminished, since in the first few years of Barrio Adentro's existence the doctors had attended to afflictions that had gone untreated for years. Over time, the most pressing primary care needs were diminishing; thus it was possible for one physician to serve an area once served by two, or for medical personnel to serve larger areas than before.

6. The Cuban supply of doctors was not endless; many chose to return home after their two-year voluntary rotations were completed, and others who wanted to continue foreign missions were needed for Cuba's growing medical commitments to other countries. In 2006, for instance, some of the most experienced veterans were needed in Bolivia, which rapidly became the site of Cuba's second-largest foreign mission with over 2,000 medical personnel.

All of these shortcomings are not so surprising given the ad hoc nature of this massive medical program, but the necessary adjustments probably could have been made if not for the difficulty of implementing central government directives in a way that efficiently serves the active participants at the grassroots neighborhood level. Barrio Adentro's biggest problems have stemmed from an affliction common to many social missions in Venezuela, one accurately diagnosed by the Bolivarian Society of General Comprehensive Medicine's Dr. Delgado, who cited the weakness of regional and state bureaucrats: "In ninety percent of cases they have been ineffective." Because Venezuela still suffers from a bureaucratic sickness that has plagued it for many decades, Chávez inherited an incomprehensible maze of useless offices from previous presidencies and state governments, and the proliferation of more public programs tended to magnify the problem. There are few efficient, straightforward models of public and civil administration in Venezuela, so it is not surprising that in many parts of the country the offices charged with coordinating the medical and social missions at the local level were incompetent, inattentive, or corrupt. Fortunately the emerging structures of participatory democracy, as embodied in the neighborhood health committees and community councils have often been able to bring these inefficiencies to light. Still, building coherent networks of responsibility and authority that draw strength from these grassroots democratic bodies remains one of the biggest challenges for the Bolivarian Revolution.

Counterrevolutionary Attempts
to Disrupt the Medical Missions

A group of disaffected Venezuelans and Cuban exiles began to actively encourage Cuban medical personnel to desert their foreign missions as soon as Barrio Adentro was established. In 2004, a small organization in Miami called Solidarity Without Borders cooperated with members of the political opposition in Venezuela to create an organization called Barrio Afuera, meaning "out of the neighborhood." *El Universal,* one of the major opposition newspapers in Caracas, ran a story in 2004 about "Cuban doctors escaping with the aid of a Venezuelan network, Barrio Afuera."

One Cuban who responded to Barrio Afuera was Otto Sanchez, a doctor who arrived in Venezuela in October of 2003. He then conspired to leave the country with the help of opposition supporters who provided him with free lodging and support in Venezuela until the U.S. embassy approved his defection to Miami. Sanchez told reporters he was unhappy to be sent to Venezuela and used for a "political program." He also complained about the pay: "You realize that you're being exploited with the kind of salary you're paid." As it turned out, these reasons were a pretext. Sanchez later revealed that he had intended to escape from his obligations long before he arrived in Venezuela because he had been a member of a small anti-government group for years in Cuba. His cousin, a member of the same dissident group, had gone into exile years earlier and was one of the founders of the Solidarity Without Borders organization in Miami.

Although a small number of medical personnel did leave their Barrio Adentro posts over the next few years, the Bush administration tried to boost the level of defection in 2006. In an exceptionally cynical effort to disrupt the Cuban humanitarian missions, not just in Venezuela but all over the world, the United States instituted the Cuban Medical Professional Parole Program. The policy allowed Cuban doctors, nurses, administrators, lab technicians, sports trainers, and other people loosely associated with the humanitarian medical missions to visit the host country's U.S. embassy and apply for quick and easy entry into the United States. Once they arrived in the United States, exile organizations like Solidarity Without Borders and other groups in Miami promised to help support the deserters. Julie M. Feinsilver, a U.S. expert on Cuban health care and medical internationalism, wrote that the Bush administration had recognized "the political and economic benefit to Cuba of its medical diplomacy program" and decided "to thwart it by offering fast-track asylum to Cuban doctors providing medical aid in third world countries."[16]

A *Wall Street Journal* article written by an anti-Castro Cuban American in August of 2010 reported that according to the Department of Homeland Security nearly 1,500 Cuban medical personnel entered the United States between 2006 and 2010 under the "parole" program. This seems to have been a gross exaggeration, about three times the number cited in cables from the U.S. embassy in Caracas that were released by WikiLeaks in 2010.[17] Another news account based on interviews with anti-Castro Cuban exiles in Miami claimed in a headline that "Almost 500 Cuban Doctors Defected to the U.S.," while the article correctly reports that 500 was the approximate number of defections by all those working in health care–related fields. Though the figures may be inflated by prejudiced parties, even the exaggerated numbers demonstrate that defectors constitute a small percentage of those performing international missions, since the same article said that 45,000 Cuban medical personnel were working in Venezuela as of 2010. The total number of medical workers involved with Barrio Adentro since its inception would be far higher because most volunteers rotate in and out of Venezuela on two year assignments.

The idea that medical personnel, and the Cuban people in general, are being exploited as "slave labor" by "Fidel, Raul, and Hugo" is a constant theme pushed by rabidly anti-Castro websites and organizations in Miami. In February of 2010, seven doctors and one nurse brought lawsuits to a federal court in Miami claiming they had suffered terribly from "involuntary servitude" and dangerous living conditions while in Venezuela; each wanted to be rewarded $60 million in damages from the Venezuelan government, the Cuban government, and PDVSA, the state-owned oil company of Venezuela.

Such over-the-top media performances orchestrated by Cuban-American lawyers are unlikely to succeed, nor do they have much effect on the huge majority of Cuban volunteers who continue to take pride in their missions. Larry Birns, director of the Council on Hemispheric Affairs in Washington, told the *South Florida Sun Sentinel* that other Cubans look at defecting doctors "as having sold out for the most craven of reasons." And according to Leonardo Hernandez, a young Cuban doctor who worked in rural Venezuela, this amounts to more than desertion from national duty, for it is also an abandonment of one's personal integrity. When an Associated Press reporter asked for his reaction to the deserters, he replied, "It's like betraying oneself as a doctor, as a person. What we're doing here is something too beautiful to stop."[18]

Some individual deserters were marginal to the medical professions, like Beny Alfonso Rodriguez, a twenty-three-year-old who was supposed to coordinate food, lodging, and transportation for a group of Cuban doctors arriving in a Venezuelan town. Rodriguez told reporters he had joined the mission with the firm intention of fleeing from service once he arrived in Venezuela. "I was born into the revolution," he said, "but I didn't choose it."[19] With help from Venezuelans who oppose Chávez, Rodriguez packed some clothes, stuffed about $600 in his pocket and was on his way to the Colombian border. He made his way to Bogotá where he applied for "parole" at the U.S. embassy and was approved within a month. Once in Miami he was offered a job delivering pizzas at night.

Although the U.S. media and Cuban exile blogs have suggested that growing numbers of Cubans working in various capacities in Venezuela are being lured away from the assignments, it is not clear that the "parole" program increased the rate of desertion among health professionals. The Cuban government has known for many years that it would lose a certain number of volunteers; for the most part, these are people who are tempted by richer lifestyles than they can enjoy in austere Cuba, or who develop love relationships in foreign countries. The 2006 documentary film *Salud*,[20] which gives an impressive overview of Cuban medical missions and medical training, reveals that a steady percentage, about 2 percent of all medical volunteers, have chosen not to return to their home island. Two doctors who are interviewed in the film reveal that they stayed behind in South Africa to get married and set up lucrative private practices, and the filmmakers illustrate the point by talking to one doctor as he arrives at his lavish home in his big Mercedes-Benz.

These kinds of doctors are outnumbered many times over by Cuban doctors who have liked their foreign assignments so much that they have signed up for second, third, and fourth missions to other countries. In addition, the supply of new doctors who are available to go on their revolutionary missions keeps increasing and helps Cuba meet new commitments that would be daunting, if not impossible, for any other nation to contemplate. When problems with Barrio Adentro were rectified in the fall of 2009 so that no neighborhood consulting offices remained unoccupied, it was because 1,000 fresh Cuban doctors were immediately available to go to Venezuela as reinforcements. One of them, Dr. Lejany Galano, who arrived on October 8, 2009, the forty-second anniversary of Che's death, told Venezuelan reporters, "Just as Che Guevara gave his life for the Latin American cause, we Cuban doctors are ready to do the same. . . . We Cuban doctors devote everything to love and solidarity, because that's what we have been taught since we were little, in school, that Che Guevara is the best example of internationalism."[21]

This intrepid spirit has been noted by Australian surgeon Katharine Edyvane, who has worked on international aid projects that are funded by the Australian government in East Timor, the small island whose society was devastated in its battle for independence from Indonesia. Over the years, she has met many Cuban doctors whom she praises for their medical expertise and dedication, while also noting that some have to endure especially lonely assignments and hardships: "One 25-year-old GP had lived and worked for the last two years in a mountain village eight hours' walk from the hospital. . . . He lived in a small room attached to the clinic, with electricity for only four hours in the evening—which meant there was no fan or air-conditioning for the oppressive tropical heat overnight, no screens for insects other than a mosquito net over the bed, and no television."[22]

The Cuban doctors who come to East Timor, noted Dr. Edyvane, have the same motivations that bring their colleagues to Venezuela, Latin America, and Africa: the desire to see different parts of the world and different cultures; the humanitarian dedication to help those who are suffering; the opportunity to develop as clinicians because they are treating maladies that one would never see in Cuba; and finally, the chance to earn a little extra money, usually a few hundred dollars a month that is often used to buy electronic equipment and cameras that are very expensive in Cuba. Still, Dr. Edyvane acknowledged, there were a few doctors who chose not to return home when their missions were completed in East Timor: nine out of 302.

Thus it appears that the U.S. State Department's "parole" program and related media efforts have failed to discourage Cuban medical workers and derail the international medical missions. These activities are notable because they demonstrate not only the United States' determination to disrupt the Cuban initiatives by any means necessary, but also the depth of Washington's concern about the democratic revolutionary movements that are sprouting up in the Western Hemisphere. For all the boastful talk from the United States and its conservative allies in Latin America about the superiority of globalizing capitalism, they are resorting to sabotage because they cannot compete with the new ideas and practices that are being generated by the new approaches to socialism that are appearing in the twenty-first century.

10. The Battle of Ideas and the Battle for Our America

> We send doctors, not soldiers!
> —FIDEL CASTRO

> The battle of ideas, there is the key.
> —HUGO CHÁVEZ

> Trenches of ideas are worth more than trenches of stone.
> —JOSÉ MARTÍ

When José Martí died in 1895, Cuba was on the verge of winning its war for independence and ending four hundred years of colonization by Spain. A few years earlier, Martí had warned that Cuba and "our America" (that is, all of America south of the United States) would be facing another threat. "The scorn of our formidable neighbor who does not know us," he wrote, "is our America's greatest danger." When Spain was pushed out of the way in 1898, the colossus of the north was ready to encroach economically and politically, especially on its nearest neighbor. The United States invaded Cuba and promptly turned over its major industries, sugar and tobacco, to U.S. corporations, established a naval base at Guantánamo, and then proceeded to tolerate and encourage corrupt, brutal, and obsequious governments for the next sixty years. When the Cuban Revolution successfully ended U.S. control in 1959, the negative influence of the dangerous neighbor did not abate. The United States began a fifty-year onslaught of multi-pronged attacks—invasions, terrorist bombings, biological warfare, an extremely harsh and continuous economic blockade, and a never-ending torrent of disinformation and media sabotage.

One of the best summations of the CIA's terrorist war against Cuba during the 1960s and 1970s came from Richard Helms, CIA director for part of that period. He testified before the House Select Committee on Assassinations in 1978 about the CIA's attempts to assassinate Fidel Castro, stating that the strategy also included "invasions of Cuba which we were constantly running under government aegis. We had task forces that were striking at Cuba constantly. We were attempting to blow up power plants. We were attempting to ruin sugar mills. We were attempting to do all kinds of things in this period. This was a matter of American government policy."[1]

Since then, the scale of violent attacks has diminished greatly, although sporadic terrorist hotel bombings and attempts at assassination continued to be perpetrated by Cuban-American terrorists from Miami, who were either tolerated or encouraged by various U.S. administrations. This did not mean, however, that U.S. hatred for an independent socialist government in the hemisphere had diminished; after the fall of the Soviet Union and its allies, the United States chose to intensify the economic blockade, the diplomatic chicanery, and the media attacks aimed at Cuba.

In the first decades of the revolutionary government, Cuba's survival entailed reliance on the Soviet Union and its satellites, a process that tied Cuba into the economic and political networks of these countries. In general, Cubans kept developing their own course toward socialism, and over time imbued their society with a distinct vision of the future, strongly rooted in the historic legacy of José Martí and other Cuban patriots. This legacy helped writers such as Cintio Vitier, the renowned poet and a Catholic, remain loyal to the revolution despite grim periods like the "*el quinquenio gris*," or "five gray years" between 1971 and 1975, when Soviet influence led to cultural repression of intellectual and artistic expression. In an essay titled "Resistance and Freedom," written during the depths of the special period, Vitier explained why the Cuban nation would not succumb to even the most extreme capitalist pressures:

> The collapse of East European socialism, including the USSR, has not provoked in Cuba, in spite of the enormous economic trauma we are suffering, the ideological vacuum expected by the United States and the Cuban reactionaries who want to take control of the island again. The reason is simple: however important our alliance with the socialist countries may have been, it was no more than that: an alliance. Where they expected to find an ideological vacuum, they found Carlos Manuel de Céspedes, Antonio Maceo, and Martí—that is, something more than an ideology, a concrete vocation of justice and liberty. The Cuban national-popular interpretation of Marxist-Leninist socialism was to put it to the service of that vocation. From the first generation of Cuban Marxists, those of the twenties, it was clear that the national tradition, culminating in Martí, would not be subsidiary to Marxism; rather, the reverse. Curiously, it is this hierarchization that explains, in the sphere of our popular culture, why the ideological values of socialism have not been destroyed among us by the collapse of the above-mentioned alliance. It is not that Cubans are more Marxist than anyone else but rather that our way of assuming "what is" Marxist in the intuitive popular interpretation has those ancillary characteristics that the collapse brings out into the open and leaves intact, since they have made possible a work of justice that is visible to all and that our concrete historical vocation clamored for.[2]

The Battle of Ideas

The Cuban government survived the desperate economic situation during the special period of the 1990s by conceding space to capitalist influences and tolerating inequalities caused by the surge of dollars into the tourist industry. But decided by the end of the decade Cuba decided it was necessary to consciously rebuild the revolutionary basis of equality and solidarity in its society, and reassert the importance of socialist, humanistic values. Fidel Castro, in his May Day speech of 2000, told the Cuban people that the ability of their nation to survive and maintain its revolutionary independence depended on being willing to fight and win a "Battle of Ideas." Among other things, he emphasized that "Revolution means . . . being treated and treating others like human beings."

In the process of serving humans instead of capital, some things would have to be sacrificed, and the fantasy of reaching first world levels of material wealth was at the top of the list. In an interview with journalists Alejandro Massia and Julio Otero in 2004, Cuba's minister of culture, Abel Prieto, pointed out that Cuba could not compete with wealthy consumer societies by trying to promise every Cuban family two cars, a swimming pool, and their own vacation house. "However," he said, "we can guarantee conditions of a decent life and at the same time a rich life in spiritual and cultural terms. It is a conception of culture as a form of growth and personal realization that is related to the quality of life. In this sense, we are convinced that culture can be an antidote against consumerism and against the oft-repeated idea that only buying can create happiness in this world."[3]

In a world that seemed hell-bent on glorifying consumption and stock market values, Cuba chose to emphasize human and social development over conventional measures of capitalist economic growth, and expanded investment in health, education, while also delivering new kinds of social services. More teacher training allowed class sizes to be reduced at all levels of primary and secondary education, and the government also created new ways to inform the entire public: new television channels offered university television classes; extension courses were instituted in all municipalities of the nation; special schools were set up in the most remote rural areas; and new computer technical courses were affected as personal and office computers became available for the first time.[4]

Whereas the battle of ideas involves building socialist values and resisting capitalist encroachment, it has also required Cuba to confront the real problems that its revolution has not yet solved. In important speeches in 2005, Fidel warned that some of the most serious threats to his nation were not external, but internal, and praised thousands of young people who had been deployed to fight low-level corruption and petty theft at the state-run gas stations. And in 2010, Raul Castro and other Cuban leaders frankly admitted that the overall economy was not functioning nearly as well as it could and embarked on a large-scale reorganization of work that emphasized more initiative, ownership, and responsibility at the individual level, and less of the state paternalism that had guaranteed employment to redundant workers. The Cuban Trade Union Confederation announced that the state sector workforce would gradually be reduced by half a million people; they, in turn, would have to find self-employment or jobs in cooperative businesses and farms.

In the realm of culture, Cuba's intellectuals were encouraged to share their work with the whole island and demonstrate that revolutionary theory and art could be adapted to twenty-first century realities. At times, this effort has had a defensive character, stressing anti-imperialism (in particular, resistance to U.S. intrusions throughout the Americas and the rest of the world) and the heroism of the Cuban Five, the anti-terrorists who are imprisoned in the United States for trying to unmask the terror networks operating out of Miami. On the other hand, Cuba also celebrated the alternatives to capitalist globalization in the form of socialist internationalism, and was ready to assert itself as an international force, not in the military sense, but in terms of trying to demonstrate that Cuba could take its ideas out into the developing world, where they could be welcomed and adapted to the needs of the people, especially in Latin America.

In this context, Cuba has developed medical and educational brigades that are fighting disease and illiteracy, efforts that are in stark contrast with the emphasis on military intervention and the ruthless exploitation of mineral resources still favored by the developed capitalist world. Cuba, as a small country, does not have the potential to help other nations resist capitalism by force, but it does have the capacity to act as a model for others who have not benefited from capitalist patterns of development over the past five hundred years. In this sense, Cuban identity is suffused with a strong international component that was suggested by José Martí over a century ago, when he wrote, *"Patria es humanidad"*—"The fatherland is all humanity." Abel Prieto has explained why this renewal process was so important, not just for Cuba, but for the world:

> In contrast to the stupidity, barbarity and the law of the strongest that today intends to impose itself worldwide, we try to defend the idea that another world is possible. We believe that what should be globalized are not bombs or hatred but peace, solidarity, health, education for all, culture, et cetera. That is why, when our physicians go to help in other countries, although their mission is to work for medical attention, they are also bearers of our values and our ideas of solidarity. This is the essence of the Battle of Ideas.[5]

Why Venezuela Joins the Battle

In 1948, Venezuela's most famous novelist, Romulo Gallegos, the country's first democratically elected president, won the support of 73 percent of the voters. They were enthusiastic about his government's plans to collect 50 percent of all oil revenues, redistribute some of the unused farmland of the very rich to the poor, and end the Church's dominance over education. These proposals were not welcomed by the local oligarchy, the Rockefeller oil interests, the Catholic Church, and the leading Venezuelan generals, so Gallegos was removed by a military coup after only eight months in office. The president believed the U.S. government was involved, either directly or indirectly, in his downfall, although this has never been proven conclusively. But certainly the United States was happy with the situation, just as it was with the coup d'états in Iran and Guatemala a few years later, where there is a clear historical record of the orchestration of events in the written documents of the CIA and the U.S. State Department.

A half century later, another Venezuelan president, Hugo Chávez, began to talk about harnessing oil revenues, redistributing land to the poor, and rebuilding the education and health systems on behalf of the majority. When Venezuela signed agreements of cooperation with Cuba in 2000 and 2001 and enlisted Cuban expertise in reforming its systems of education and medicine, the U.S. government, multinational oil corporations, the Venezuelan oligarchy, and the Catholic Church hierarchy all agreed that Hugo Chávez was a grave threat to the Western Hemisphere. But this time, unlike 1948, the military coup d'état was not successful. While the U.S. State Department tried to deny involvement in the coup, its own Office of Inspector General found otherwise several months later when it reported: "It is clear that NED, Department of Defense (DOD), and other U.S. assistance programs provided training, institution building, and other support to individuals and organizations understood to be actively involved in the brief ouster of the Chávez government."[6]

While seeking to sabotage the budding Bolivarian Revolution and bury the incredibly persistent Cuban Revolution, the United States revealed the paucity of ideas that was afflicting the center of the advanced capitalist world. Hugo Chávez noticed this lack of underlying philosophical confidence, and in his characteristically bold fashion, announced that it was time for those opposed to capitalist globalization to go on the offensive. At the Meeting of Artists and Intellectuals in Defense of Humanity, a wide array of left-leaning people from the Americas and other parts of the world who came to Caracas in late 2004, he declared that it was not sufficient for those who work in the realm of ideas and the imagination to defend humanistic values. It was also necessary, he said, to go on the offensive in the sense of enhancing humanistic values and demonstrating that "another world" was indeed possible. At the conclusion of this meeting, on December 5, 2004, Chávez said, "It is necessary to review the history of socialism and rescue the concept of socialism." And on January 30, 2005, at the World Social Forum, he added, "We have to reinvent socialism. It can't be the kind of socialism we saw in the Soviet Union." Then, at the Social Debt Summit, February 25, 2005, Chávez publicly announced for the first time that the task lying ahead was to "invent twenty-first-century socialism," a term that had been used first by Chilean sociologist Tomas Moulian about five years earlier.[7]

The idea of North American imperialism threatening Latin America did not spring into Chávez's head because he had been brainwashed by Cubans, but because his Bolivarian Revolutionary Movement, established in 1982 among progressive young army officers, was directly descended from the thinking of Simon Bolívar, Venezuela's national hero. After he liberated half of South America from the imperial rule of the Spanish, Bolívar had warned: "The United States of America seems to be destined by providence to condemn [our] America to misery in the name of Liberty." Furthermore, when Chávez identified the Venezuelan oligarchy as the internal enemy, he was not merely referring to their twentieth-century collusion with international capitalism and their backing of the coup to depose him in 2002. He was expressing the visceral feeling that had been deeply ingrained in the country's oppressed majority for centuries, best expressed by Ezequiel Zamora, another Venezuelan hero, who led an army of campesinos and slaves in the Federal Wars of the 1850s and 1860s, and called for "free elections, free land and free men, horror to the oligarchy."

ALBA and the Prospect for Change

Cuba and Venezuela could not have embarked on their ambitious projects over the last decade without the increasing cooperation of other countries in Latin America. Some large nations such as Brazil and Argentina, and smaller countries such as Chile and Uruguay, had center-left leaders who did not push very far to the left in their domestic endeavors but did extend international diplomatic solidarity to Cuba and Venezuela. They joined with other nations within the growing circle of UNASUR, MERCOSUR, and other hemispheric bodies to help shield the more revolutionary societies from the attacks mounted by the United States. Brazil, in particular, was willing and able to engage in many practical large-scale economic and social projects that benefited both Venezuela and Cuba, and sheltered them to some extent from subversive economic and political strategies of the United States. These natives admired Fidel Castro and Hugo Chávez, and felt indebted to them, too, because they had demonstrated that it was possible to stand up to imperial pressure and still survive in the Western Hemisphere, thus allowing the rest of the Americas to assert, even though in milder ways, their own independence.

The most significant movement toward international cooperation in the Western Hemisphere has come through the formation of ALBA, the Bolivian Alliance of the Peoples of Our America (from 2005 until 2009 it was called the Bolivarian Alternative for the Peoples of Our America). The words "Our America" in the name of the organization echo the title of one of José Martí's most famous essays, in which he developed the concept of a larger America that does not permit itself to be bullied and controlled by the United States. The membership of ALBA does not add up to a formidable rival of the United States, for by 2009 it only consisted of five rather small countries—Cuba, Venezuela, Bolivia, Ecuador, Honduras, and Nicaragua—and the tiny island nations of Dominica, Antigua and Barbuda, Saint Vincent, and the Grenadines. Collectively, the strength of these nations paled beside the United States, for they had a combined population of about 75 million, only one-quarter of that of the United States, and a combined Gross Domestic Product of about $650 billion, less than 5 percent of the $14.5 trillion GDP generated annually in the United States.[8] (The ALBA numbers diminished somewhat in 2010, when a military coup removed Honduras, with its 8 million people and it $32 billion GDP, from the equation.)

The ALBA countries are cooperating with one another, each one with politics defined within its own nationalistic context, each with its own social and cultural goals linked to twenty-first-century socialism. The concrete measures they are pursuing are being implemented in part by gaining control over the development and sale of natural resources in order to promote more social spending and social equality. These progressive actions by the ALBA governments have nothing in common with Soviet-style mass expropriations of the means of industrial and agricultural production, and they do not utilize secret police or any other kind of state coercion. In fact, a great many of the social, political, and economic policies that they are putting into practice are not so different than those undertaken under the New Deal in the United States or by the social democratic governments of Europe during the twentieth century. The kinds of changes implemented include the provision of free education for all and the elimination of illiteracy, the use of revenues from national resource production to help reduce poverty, the pursuit of moderate land reform, more efficient and honest collection of taxes, the expansion of social security and pensions, general wage increases for working people, and the creation of more inclusive and universal public health systems. This is not to say that the long-term goals of the ALBA nations only consist of the social democratic amelioration of capitalist excesses, for they have also stated or implied that they will be instituting social ownership of various productive activities and introducing direct and participatory democratic control of many social institutions. Each country has also stated that it will make such changes in its own particular ways in keeping with its own national culture, leaving parts of the economy in private hands, encouraging small businesses, and respecting individual ownership of property when it does not represent a threat to social well-being.

Since Cuba and Venezuela were the original members of ALBA in 2005, they have been able to provide the most cooperative assistance to the other members. Cuba has provided most of the human capital and expert personnel in health care, education, and other fields. Venezuela has been contributing the efforts of its technicians, engineers, and other experts to the construction projects and medical installations in various nations, but has made its greatest impact with shipments of petroleum at reduced prices, or by giving outright grants and interest-free loans for socially useful projects. Though this kind of helpful diplomacy is labeled by critics as a form of "buying political support," it is actually similar to aid packages put together by wealthy capitalist countries except for one important proviso—Venezuela does not attach commercial tie-ins or obligations. Many wealthy nations, including the United States, have constructed aid programs that actively promote entrée for their own multinational manufacturing and extractive corporations. Venezuela, though not nearly as rich as those capitalist nations, is wealthier than most developing nations, and is trying to demonstrate how a large state producer of natural resources can share the proceeds of resource extraction, or in this case, the oil itself, more fairly with those nations and poor populations that lack such resources and are at a distinct disadvantage in the world market. The ALBA nations have even developed their own currency, the *sucre*, which is calculated electronically to facilitate large-scale exchanges of goods among members under fair terms uninfluenced by the fluctuations of the world commodity or currency markets. If ALBA nations can withstand the increasingly harsh political and economic reaction from the United States, they will likely attract even more members in the Western Hemisphere.

Nicaragua and Bolivia:
Breaking Free from Neoliberalism

Long before ALBA, and two full decades before Cuban medical missions went to Venezuela, Cuba was helping to build new primary medical care and educational systems in another Latin American country. As soon as the Sandinista Revolution managed to overthrow the Somoza dictatorship in Nicaragua in 1979, Cuban doctors traveled there to assist in the formation of rural and urban clinics that served the poor. The Sandinistas can be seen as forerunners of those who are constructing twenty-first-century socialism, for they were attempting to fashion a distinctive brand of revolution appropriate to their particular history and culture. Three of the key ingredients were a strong nationalist identification with the democratic and egalitarian goals of their guerrilla hero, Augusto Sandino; a positive faith in the theology of liberation that at the time in Latin America was changing the Catholic Church (and the government, too, since three out of seven members of the Sandinista leadership were priests); and an evolving mix of progressive and Marxist ideas that were quite distinct from old Soviet socialist models.

Shortly after the Sandinistas took power it was estimated that 300 of the 1,300 Nicaraguan doctors that had been practicing medicine had left the country. This was soon remedied by the arrival of approximately 850 foreign doctors, many of them sympathetic medical professionals from Europe, Canada, and the United States, but the majority from Cuba. The increase in personnel was timely because it allowed the new government to rapidly expand its primary health program: in 1977 there were 172 health centers nationwide and by 1982 there were 429, and another 37 were scheduled to be constructed in 1983. Health care expenditures had risen from 3 percent of the national budget to 11 percent. In terms of health outcomes, the *Canadian Medical Association Journal* reported that between 1978 and 1983, infant mortality decreased from 121 to 80.2 per 1,000 live births, and life expectancy at birth rose from fifty-two to fifty-nine years.[9]

Another momentous change in the early years of the Sandinista government was the expansion in medical education. Less than five years after the Sandinista triumph there were ten times more students studying to be physicians (900), and Cuban professors were assisting in instruction; six times as many students were training to become registered nurses; and three times as many people were studying to be nurse's aides.

Cuban education experts also helped in primary and secondary schools after brigades of Nicaraguan high school and college students had spread out through the country to teach the illiterate majority how to read and write. In less than a decade, their efforts dramatically reduced the illiteracy rate from 52 to 12 percent.

All of this was bad news to the Reagan administration in Washington, which claimed that the whole operation was being orchestrated by Cuban terrorists, who in turn were agents of the

Soviet Union. The United States spent the entire decade of the 1980s trying to undermine the Sandinistas' efforts to improve the economic and social reality of the Nicaraguan population, imposing a crushing economic embargo and launching a lethal counterrevolutionary war. The Contras, the counterrevolutionary forces created by the CIA, took particular pleasure in destroying public health outposts and schools and intimidating health workers and teachers. In 1983, just four years after the triumph of the revolution, "16 health workers, including one French and one German physician, have been killed, 27 others have been seriously wounded, and 30 have been kidnapped and tortured along the country's northern border. In addition, three health educators, seven medical students, and at least 40 health volunteers have been killed by the contras. At least two hospitals and 19 health centers and posts have been destroyed."[10] Furthermore, the construction plans for more than half of the health posts had to be abandoned because of the attacks along the nation's borders with Honduras and Costa Rica.

Several years of constant military and economic battering finally exhausted all Nicaraguans to the extent that opposition political forces, openly backed and financed by the United States, won the 1990 elections. The Sandinistas peacefully relinquished power to the conservative victors, who dutifully followed U.S. free market guidelines and instructions from the U.S. embassy for the next seventeen years. One would think that the United States, if only to enhance its own image during that period of time, would have allocated a little money to ameliorative social measures so that ordinary Nicaraguans lived a little more decently.

That was not the case. The return to conservative, free market rule was characterized by social neglect, and was clearly disastrous for most Nicaraguans. By 2007 their country had the highest rate of malnutrition in Central America, and 80 percent of the people lived in poverty, 45 percent in absolutely destitute conditions. Illiteracy had nearly tripled over the decade and a half of pro-U.S. rule, largely because neoliberal policies meant there were not sufficient government revenues to continue the Sandinista commitment to free education for all

children; an astounding 800,000 children (Nicaragua's total population was only 6 million) were not going to school by 2007.[11]

That year the Sandinistas were able to win back the presidency
despite heavy diplomatic and financial opposition from the north and
a political campaign orchestrated by the U.S. embassy that emphasized the danger of Hugo Chávez, whom they accused of intending
(with Cuban help, of course) to take over Nicaragua. The Sandinistas,
who won in spite of this interference, were happy to accept Cuban
humanitarian aid, for immediately after their victory, they once again
launched a literacy program, this time utilizing the Cuban "Yo, Si
Puedo" (Yes, I Can) system, which had already been successfully
employed in the fight against illiteracy in Venezuela and Bolivia. In
just two years, by 2009, UNESCO announced that Nicaragua was, by
their standards, "free of illiteracy," meaning that the rate had fallen
below 4 percent. Simultaneously, educational opportunities expanded
for hundreds of thousands of Nicaraguan schoolchildren who had
been excluded from public education because of extreme poverty;
they began attending school regularly because the government eliminated all public school fees and then instituted a program of free meals
for all who needed them. In addition, the Sandinistas also declared
that once again free health care would be provided to the entire population and utilized help from Cuba, Venezuela, and ALBA to build
and equip sixteen new hospitals and high-tech clinics.

The new alliances and the reconfiguration of social, political, and
economic forces in the Western Hemisphere that had allowed
Nicaragua to get back on a progressive course were also important in
supporting Bolivia's political emergence in 2006 after Evo Morales
was elected president. The United States reacted negatively, but not
simply because Morales and Bolivia joined ALBA a few months after
the election. Long before Morales became the first indigenous leader
to rule his country in five centuries, the United States had identified
him and his social and political organization, MAS (Movimiento al
Socialismo), as the most threatening challenger to the neoliberal pres-
idential candidates that Washington was backing. The U.S. ambassador in 2002, Manual Rocha, took the aggressive step of publicly

warning the Bolivian people not to vote for Morales, thinking that he could frighten voters by suggesting that the candidate's support for impoverished coca farmers meant that he also was in league with international drug syndicates: "As a representative of the United States, I want to remind the Bolivian electorate that if you elect those who want Bolivia to become a major cocaine exporter again, this will endanger the future of U.S. assistance to Bolivia." Even though Morales failed to win that election, it was not because of the ambassador's interference; most political observers inside Bolivia felt that Evo's popularity was enhanced by this kind of crude interference.

Bolivia, like Nicaragua and Venezuela, has begun constructing a socialist identity of its own in keeping with its national history. Evo Morales and his administration confidently talked about moving toward a distinctly Bolivian kind of twenty-first-century socialism, a "communitarian socialism" built around ancient indigenous values of sharing and community labor. Included in this vision was a strong concern for protecting Pachamama, or Mother Earth, from global warming and other environmental threats. The Bolivian leader stressed the idea of "living well" instead of "living better," meaning that citizens should reject the capitalist/consumerist urge to compete to see who amasses more possessions, and instead create a society in which all people live in dignity, leading modest and sufficient material lives that are in harmony with nature.

The idea of socialism built on communitarian, indigenous traditions is not new to the Andean nations. Early in the twentieth century, Peruvian revolutionary and theorist José Carlos Mariátegui insisted that the European models for revolution would not be appropriate for South America, and proposed building a kind of "natural socialism" that would expand the revolutionary project beyond the urban working class to include the impoverished, laboring masses in the countryside: "In Peru those masses are four-fifths indigenous. Thus our socialism must declare its solidarity with the native people."[12] "Certainly, we do not wish that socialism in America be a tracing and a copy. It must be a heroic creation. We must, with our own reality, in our own language, bring Indoamerican socialism to life."[13] One contemporary Bolivian indigenous writer, Marcelo Saavedra Vargas, says that the indigenous people have an interpretation of "materialism" that is wholly different than the rampant overconsumption practiced by the so-called materialistic nations of the north. "It is capitalist society that rejects materialism. It makes war on the material world and destroys it. We, on the other hand, embrace the material world, consider ourselves part of it, and care for it."[14]

As soon as Evo Morales took office in 2006, Bolivians knew that they must enhance the education of the poor if they were going to construct a different kind of society. They immediately employed the Cuban "Yo, Si Puedo" literacy program, with the result that one and a half million illiterate people were taught to read in the next two years. At the end of 2008, UNESCO declared that the nation was free of illiteracy. In the meantime, the government had initiated a number of related efforts to help students who had reached the first stages of literacy continue their studies. By 2010, new programs and incentives had enabled one million people to study toward a fifth-grade level of education.

Since Bolivia elected to become the third member of ALBA in 2006, it availed itself of the opportunity to improve health care and bring free medical services to the poor. In the first year, in addition to bringing over 2,000 Cuban medical personnel to provide primary care in underserved areas, ALBA agreements provided 5,000 scholarships for Bolivian students to study medicine in Cuba. Venezuelan engineering teams arrived to help build numerous hospitals and polyclinics, as well as the surgical centers for Mission Milagro, which then proceeded to perform over 500,000 eye operations over the next four years. Interestingly, nearly 100,000 of these patients were poor residents of Brazil, Peru, Paraguay, and Argentina who eagerly crossed their borders with Bolivia to find the nearest eye clinic that could offer them free surgery and medical care.

The United States, of course, was taking note of these successes and trying to strengthen the local opposition. When Cuban doctors started treating the impoverished Bolivian majority, there were negative responses from local elites and protests from the Bolivian medical association that were similar to defamatory campaigns mounted in Venezuela and other parts of the Americas. They either disparaged Cuban doctors as inept, unqualified practitioners who could only disrupt health care delivery or portrayed them as immensely clever political/military agents who would brainwash the public with communist propaganda. Within a few months, as word of the quality of care circulated among grassroots communities, this kind of criticism dissipated. It was followed in some areas, such as the wealthy department of Santa Cruz, by direct actions by right-wing political forces that were assisted in their anti-government and separatist activities by officials and contractors of the U.S. State Department. Some with violent tendencies, emboldened by this support, decided to mount physical attacks on Cuban medical personnel.[15] In August of 2008, members of the ultra-right-wing Civic Comité and Unión Juvenil Cruceñista (the Santa Cruz Union of Youth) kidnapped a number of Cuban medical personnel from a residence they occupied in Santa Cruz, beat them and threatened to kill them, forced them into a pickup truck, drove them ten kilometers into the countryside, dumped them on the side of the road, and warned them to return to Cuba if they wanted to stay alive.[16] These kinds of incidents, including many violent racist attacks against indigenous citizens, did not have the success they had in Nicaragua in the 1980s.   Instead, they motivated President Evo Morales to act more forcefully against the insurrectionist movement in the state of Santa Cruz and take action against the U.S. ambassador in La Paz, Philip Goldberg, who had been holding meetings with the separatists. He was expelled from Bolivia in September of 2008.

Honduras and Haiti: No Escaping U.S. Influence

Not every ALBA story has been a happy one, for as fragile as Nicaragua's new independence has been, other countries in Central America and the Caribbean such as Honduras and Haiti are even more vulnerable to intervention from the north. It is remarkable that Honduras, which has been dominated by a U.S. diplomatic and military presence ever since the Central American wars of the 1980s, was able to join ALBA even for a short time, from 2007 until 2009. This occurred during the presidency of Manuel Zelaya, a wealthy rancher and timber entrepreneur whose background in the Liberal Party did not seem to qualify him as a politician of the center-left, let alone as a revolutionary. Certainly Honduras, a country with a large U.S. Air Force base, its own entrenched armed forces well schooled in right-wing fealty to the north, and a dominant oligarchy presiding over an impoverished majority, was not a likely candidate for socialist transformation. President Zelaya, with the backing of active social movements at the grassroots level, was nevertheless able to push forward with a number of meaningful reforms. This happened because ALBA was willing to lend practical assistance to Honduras, and also because the ferment stirred up by the battle of ideas and various conceptions of twenty-first-century socialism were leading common people to believe that change, even if it was incremental, was possible. ALBA grants and low-interest loans funded rural development and agriculture, as well as supporting health, education, and technological programs. Favorable prices for petroleum purchased through Venezuela's Petrocaribe program allowed the Honduran government to free up money for social purposes, such as an initiative to make public education absolutely free for all children.

At first some of these changes were welcomed or tolerated by Zelaya's Liberal Party and many others among the elite classes, and the Congress was willing to vote for both the Petrocaribe oil agreement and the membership in ALBA in 2008. As discussed earlier in chapter 3, the Honduran Medical Association went so far as to abandon its hostile stance toward Cuban doctors and actually joined President Zelaya in ceremonies celebrating Cuban collaboration on new Honduran medical projects, such as the opening of a hospital in the remote Garifuna area by doctors who had graduated from the Latin American Medical School in Havana. Luther Castillo, the first Garifuna graduate and founder of the hospital, was named Honduran Doctor of the Year in 2007 by the International Rotary Club in the capital, Tegucigalpa.

Unfortunately, this upper-class recognition of the value of cooperation with Cuba and Venezuela lasted only briefly, until the summer of 2009, when the Honduran oligarchy and military, with the help of Cuban exiles in Miami and increasingly alarmed right-wing allies in the U.S. military, the State Department, and Washington think tanks, engineered a coup against President Zelaya. In the aftermath, when soldiers and police were violently suppressing civil society protests against the coup, they also harassed medical staff at the Garifuna hospital and threatened to close it down. Dr. Luther Castillo, as a supporter of President Zelaya, had to go into hiding to escape persecution and was forced to abandon the country. In 2010 he still could not return home, so he served as the coordinator of the first large contingent of ELAM graduates that joined the Henry Reeve Brigade and rushed to Haiti to serve as medical volunteers after the earthquake.

If the success of political experimentation was unlikely in Honduras, it was even more difficult to accomplish in Haiti a few years earlier. At the very moment that the Sandinista Revolution was nearly extinguished by the United States at the beginning of the 1990s, another revolutionary situation had begun developing in Haiti, except in this case there was no rebel army to overwhelm the corrupt military and redistribute the economic power held by a tiny elite. What Haiti had in common with Nicaragua was the development of an intense popular political movement of the impoverished majority based on liberation theology. Their organization, Fanmi Lavalas, led by parish priests such as Jean Bertrand Aristide who had been living among the poor, engaged the support of the huge majority of Haitians. In 1990, two-thirds of the voters chose Aristide as their president, but unfortunately at a time when no other countries in the hemisphere were in a position to aid a government that wanted to practice "a preferential option for the poor" preached by Aristide. With encouragement from the conservative U.S. administration under the first president Bush, corrupt military officers had little difficulty removing Aristide from power eight months later in 1991. The brutality of this regime was so widespread that the Clinton administration intervened with U.S. soldiers in 1994 and restored Aristide to the presidency, but with onerous conditions. Aristide and those who succeeded him in government had to agree to arrangements with the IMF and the World Bank that seemed to preclude progressive legislation that would help the poor. However, after Aristide was returned to the presidency by a huge majority of over 90 percent in 2000, the Haitian government was able to make some serious commitments toward social change in spite of the severe limitations imposed by the international financial institutions, the United States, France, and Canada. In 2001, Aristide declared that 20 percent of the national budget would go to education and then launched a massive literacy campaign that summer. In February of 2003, Aristide pushed for economic reforms and doubled the minimum wage; three months later his government passed legislation prohibiting trafficking in persons and regulating child domestic labor.

By this time, Cuba and Venezuela were beginning to cooperate in bilateral agreements of mutual aid and economic exchange with each other, but ALBA had not yet been founded, so they were not in a position to provide the wide-ranging kinds of aid that they offered to Bolivia a few years later. However, Cuba had continued to commit substantial health care resources to Haiti ever since its medical brigades arrived under the Comprehensive Health Plan in December 1998. At the time, there were fewer than 2,000 doctors practicing in Haiti, and 90 percent of them practiced in the cities. The Cuban presence had a substantial impact during the first three years; by June of 2002, 1,452 medical collaborators had served in Haiti and medical statistics improved dramatically in the areas where the Cuban doctors were practicing (about three-quarters of the country). For example, while fifty-nine out of 1,000 babies had died at birth in 2000, by 2002 the mortality rate was reduced to thirty-three per thousand. [17]

By 2003, health care prospects looked even brighter, for in addition to the more than 300 Haitians studying medicine at the Latin American School of Medicine in Havana, there were another 200 medical students enrolled at a brand-new university built in Port au Prince with the aid of the government of Taiwan and staffed by medical professors provided by Cuba. Even though ALBA had not been formed and Barrio Adentro was just emerging in Venezuela, Haiti's privileged elite and their conservative backers in Washington were greatly alarmed. They quickly formed political groups like the Group of 184 and the Democratic Convergence to agitate for Aristide's downfall—"We know that US funds overtly financed the opposition," wrote Dr. Paul Farmer in 2004, and he added that these political activities seemed to be coordinated with armed rebel units who had trained on the border with the Dominican Republic and acquired U.S. weapons before launching violent attacks on the Aristide government in various Haitian towns and cities.[18]

In February 2004, with the country devolving into chaos, the United States intervened with troops, engineered a neat coup d'état by quickly removing President Aristide from the country under pretense of a "rescue," and then deposited him on the other side of the ocean, in Africa. The U.S. Marines overran the new Aristide medical school, chased out the doctors and students, and used the facility as their military headquarters. The medical school would remain closed until the spring of 2010, when, with aid and personnel supplied by ALBA, classes began once again. Simultaneously, Brazil was joining the ALBA nations to help the Haitian government build the coherent public and universal medical care system that the country had needed for so long. Luther Castillo, the Honduran doctor and ELAM graduate who was forced out of his own country by the military coup of 2009, was part of the contingent of Cuban-trained physicians arriving in Haiti after the earthquake of January 2010: "There are many needs," he said, "but the challenge of forming a health system in Haiti is a unique opportunity for us. . . . We are providing medical care, opening small clinics, as a basis for creating a model of primary health care, with health promotion and prevention heavily deployed. . . . At the same time we learn the language, history, and idiosyncrasy of this people, the moral and philosophical values, the epic struggle of this nation."

Venezuela and ALBA Help Cuba
"Climb Out of the Trenches"

The formation of ALBA not only freed Cuba from its diplomatic and economic isolation, but it has provided space for the island nation to expand its revolutionary ideas in relation to revolutionary thought developing elsewhere. This is allowing the emancipatory flavor of Cuban socialism to emerge once again from its historical roots. In 1992, Cintio Vitier, the renowned poet who was a mainstay of the Center for Martí Studies in Havana for many years, wrote an essay titled "Resistance and Freedom." In it, he named the five essential conditions for the foundation of socialism and democracy in Cuba that were identical to the great ethical principles of José Martí: 1) anti-imperialism; 2) solidarity with the poor and the oppressed; 3) formation of a republic of workers; 4) the integral exercise of self; and 5) the respect, as a kind of family honor, for the integral well-being of others. Then he added:

> The latter two [the fourth and fifth listed above] are the most difficult to put into practice in the embattled trench into which our Revolution has been increasingly forced. A trench is not a parliament. Martí himself, by saying "trenches of ideas are worth more than trenches of stone," accepted that, in the face of the enemy, ideas have to become entrenched, united for a resistance without fissures.

Certainly the battle of ideas, when it was initiated at the end of the 1990s, was intended to instill the Cuban people with pride in their society and their heroic resistance to the Empire. But it also was intended to rejuvenate revolutionary concepts and practices that had been sorely tested by the hardships of the special period, and generate an enthusiasm about the creation of new socialist ideas and projects that embody the spirit of solidarity and humanity. Vitier wrote that "a trench is not a parliament" because he knew that a trench of ideas requires vigilance and resistance, and that Cuba could not experiment with a totally open debate of all ideas (a "parliament" of ideas) because it was still too vulnerable to attacks from the Empire to climb out of the trench. But he did suggest how, over the course of the coming years, Cuba might be able to liberate itself and extricate itself from the trench.

> As we delve deeper into the challenge of the nineties, each step we take, however small it may be, has to be against an enemy and in favor of our resistance. . . . Paradoxically, we also have against us the habit of resisting the Empire, which tends to keep us firm in our conviction but also immobile, as if hypnotized by resistance. To convert resistance into the mother of a new freedom is the challenge that imposes itself on us. To meet this challenge, there is no better inspiration than the libertarian spirit of Martí.

In the first decade of the twenty-first century, Cuba has been able to start climbing out of its trench, not to surrender, but to venture into the battle of ideas fortified by having others by its side. The nations of ALBA and people in other countries that have been inspired by Cuba's resistance are contributing not only their fresh energy for the struggle, but also their own concepts of what socialism can be. Hugo Chávez, Evo Morales, Rafael Correa, and Daniel Ortega, and the women and men of their countries are generating new ideas, but they do not necessarily have the same agendas and ideas, and some of their thought is certainly not fully developed. However, nearly all of their ideas share a confidence in their people's spirit and for that reason they are not afraid to experiment with new revolutionary concepts and practices.

The progressive movements in the Americas have maintained for three decades that neoliberal globalization with free markets imposed by the United States is not only harmful to their nations but avoidable, and that "Another World Is Possible." ALBA, the acronym for the Bolivarian Alternative for the Peoples of Our America, also means "dawn" in Spanish, thus suggesting that the dawn of an alternative world is at hand.

The humanitarian health and education programs can also be viewed as a form of positive diplomacy or "public diplomacy," since one of Cuba's purposes is to develop friendly relations and trust with other countries at a time when U.S. and conservative forces are depicting it as a dangerous terrorist nation. While Cuban and Venezuelan efforts are derided by right-wing detractors, such as Cuban exiles in Miami and the political opposition in Caracas, as being "propaganda" efforts, both nations have gained considerable respect from many other countries and international organizations, not only for the very real accomplishments of their programs, but also for the generosity, dedication, and competence demonstrated by individual doctors, nurses, teachers, and technicians. In many ways, they are saying to the world, "We have our own ideas about how nations and people should treat each other," and then giving a practical demonstration. In general, Cuba and Venezuela are successfully combining aid that advertises their goodwill—positive public diplomacy—with a much deeper mission: demonstrating through their engagement at the grassroots level that their behavior and ethics are consistent with the social, cultural, and political concepts of socialist development they espouse. If, in the language of their North American critics, the Cubans and Venezuelans are "selling" something, or putting a "brand" out in the "market of ideas," then their product is *solidaridad*—human solidarity. Enrique Ubieta Gómez wrote in his book *Venezuela Rebelde: solidaridad versus dinero:*

> For the first time in Venezuela there appeared another conception of life that wasn't centered on having, but on being. The Cuban internationalist doctors were a symbol of this new conception. While the revolutionary government pushed the social missions and elevated the quality of life of the poorest, offering them health, education, and culture, and new opportunities to insert themselves in work and social life, the opposition press and television kept stimulating the desire for individualism, the hope of easy riches, the idea that the quality of life can only be sustained by the accumulation of money, by consumption, and by the idolatry of the American way of life.[19]

The only sins that the ALBA nations are committing are fighting poverty at the expense of long-entrenched elites that have close ties and business relationships with the United States, and rejecting the neoliberal mantra that has been broadcast by the United States and Britain, and required by the IMF and the World Bank. Ever since Margaret Thatcher announced TINA, There Is No Alternative, in the late 1970s, the developing world has been force-fed an economic philosophy based entirely on the glorification of free markets, the purpose being to allow Western industrial and financial corporations to further penetrate and dominate developing nations where they have significant involvement in natural resources and agricultural production, as well as transnational manufacturing. Even though these policies were disastrous for nearly all of Latin America and many other parts of the third world during the 1980s and 1990s, thirty years later the masters of global capital are still insisting that a system of open markets for all multinational corporations and banks is good for developing countries.

But now, the part of the world that Che Guevara once referred to as "America with a Capital 'A'" has a real alternative, literally with a "Capital A": La Alternativa (Alianza) Bolivariana para los Pueblos de Nuestra America. ALBA is utilizing human potential, human capital, and natural resources on a national and regional scale with an emphasis not just on social justice, but on regenerating local culture and pride. Since the Bolivarians and the other new socialists are choosing to "Build It Now" (also the title of Michael Lebowitz's book on the emergence of socialism for the twenty-first century), the ideological confrontation between the needs of capital versus the needs of human beings is unavoidable. Although not every experiment undertaken by Venezuela, Cuba, or the other ALBA nations will succeed, they are showing that many of their ideas are superior to the globalized, homogenized consumer culture offered by advanced capitalism. Consequently, ALBA is inspiring others to dream of social and economic changes that can promote healthier and more dignified lives for their people. There are even signs that nations that are solidly part of first-world capitalist political economy will notice the strategies that succeed in the "battle of ideas" and will choose to collaborate in unusual ways.

At a June 2010 press conference, Cuban Foreign Minister Bruno Rodriguez and Stephen Smith, the foreign minister of Australia, announced their intention to cooperate on joint projects in East Timor and Haiti. Smith said, "Both in the Pacific and in the Caribbean you, of course, have small island states, low income, in need of capacity building, and so, given Cuba's world-class credentials in the medical training area, given our world-class expertise in child and maternal health care, we believe that there is potential for us to work together. And that's what we're exploring."[20]

This kind of exploration of new ideas is precisely what the United States has been trying to prevent.

11. The War on Ideas:
The U.S. Counterinsurgency Campaign

In the war of ideas, it's often more effective to destroy their brand
than build up ours.

—JAMES K. GLASSMAN, Undersecretary for Public Diplomacy,

U.S. State Department

Chávez and Venezuela are developing the conceptual and physical
capability to challenge the status quo in Latin America, and to generate a "super-insurgency."

—COLONEL MAX MANWARING, Strategic Studies Institute,

U.S. Army War College

The efforts of Cuba, Venezuela, and the ALBA nations to meet social
needs, provide health care, and educate their populations are pro-
gressing, not without mistakes and miscalculations, but for the most
part with results consistent with the socialist egalitarianism and
humanistic solidarity they espouse. The United States has taken note
of the contending philosophy developing in the south, but it is not
interested in engaging in a "battle of ideas" or intellectual debate with
those whose concepts and values challenge the basic tenets of global-

izing capitalism. Instead, it employs a strategy that could be best described as a *war on ideas*, an intensive assault of disinformation meant to make sure that most people, not just in the United States but around the world, are never aware that there is an alternative to capitalist values developing in the Western Hemisphere.

In 2002 and again in the spring of 2004, shortly after more than 10,000 Cuban doctors began working in Barrio Adentro clinics in Venezuela, Washington signaled, indirectly, that it was displeased with this course of events. John Bolton, U.S. undersecretary of state in the Bush adminstration, said, "We are concerned that Cuba is developing a limited biological weapons effort," and suggested that Cuba's sophisticated medical research laboratories could soon be concocting WMD, weapons of mass destruction. Though his accusation was dismissed as ridiculous by foreign policy experts, his words did have a clear purpose: the U.S. government was escalating its long-standing hostility toward Cuba because nearly a half century of attempts to isolate, intimidate, and impoverish the island were failing. Bolton was engaging in *negative branding*, a practice that would be applied with increased intensity, not only to Cuba but to all progressive forces in the hemisphere over the next several years.

James K. Glassman, who served as the undersecretary of state for public diplomacy in the Bush administration in 2008, gave a succinct description of this approach. Glassman, who referred to himself as the "regional commander in the war of ideas,"[1] told reporter Spencer Ackerman, "In the war of ideas it's often more effective to destroy their brand than build up ours." The primary task, as he put it, was "tarnishing the brand of U.S. enemies."[2] Over the past three decades, the U.S. State Department, the Department of Defense, and the CIA, as well as the corporate contractors that all three government entities employ, have attacked the ideological enemy with weapons honed for "information warfare," "strategic information," and "perception management." The terminology and rhetoric are mainly derived from two sources, the negative advertising strategies of U.S. political campaigns and the disinformation assaults perfected by military experts in PSYOP, or psychological operations.

As Cuba and Venezuela have proceeded with their ambitious programs of collaboration in medicine and other areas, the United States has increased its efforts to discredit and destabilize both nations. In order to distract attention from Cuban medical expertise and humanitarian efforts, top U.S.military and civilian leaders spread derogatory messages that are not as specific nor as easy to refute as Bolton's WMD accusation. They suggested that Cuba and Venezuela are threats to democracy and somehow linked to global terrorism. In 2004, General James Hill, commander of the U.S. military Southern Command, or SouthCom, informed Congress that the "emerging threat" to "national security" in the Western Hemisphere was the "authoritarianism" of Hugo Chávez, who was guilty of espousing a "radical populism in which the democratic process is undermined." General Craddock, who succeeded General Hill as SouthCom chief, told the U.S. Senate that the U.S. military needed to expand its role in the hemisphere in order to "prosecute the war on terrorism," "enhance regional security cooperation to counter transnational threats," and "closely coordinate in assisting partner nations' efforts to address the threats they face in maintaining effective democracies."[3] The next year, U.S. secretary of state Condoleezza Rice followed the generals' lead and warned that the Chávez government posed a "major threat to the whole region" and that the United States "cannot remain indifferent to what Venezuela is doing beyond its borders." According to one military theorist working within the SouthCom network, President Chávez of Venezuela, aided and abetted by Cuba, was a new kind of super-enemy, an expert in "asymmetrical" and "fourth- generation warfare" who was mounting a "super insurgency" campaign designed to upset the established order of the entire hemisphere. In response, according to this analysis, the Department of Defense along with the entire U.S. foreign relations and spy apparatus were going to have to mobilize new kinds of sophisticated counterinsurgency forces to destroy the threat.[4]

The Military Industrial
Diplomatic Academic Complex

It is true that Venezuela is actively influencing many people throughout the hemisphere, but only in peaceful ways that hardly could be construed as transnational threats linked to global terrorism. In early 2005, President Chávez was introducing the idea of democratic transition to "twenty-first-century socialism" at the World Social Forum in Brazil. Cuba was continuing to send medical personnel and technical advisers to many developing countries, and Venezuela was making large-scale contributions to humanitarian and economic aid projects because world oil prices were high. In 2007, Venezuela announced $8.87 billion in aid commitments to other nations in the hemisphere, none of which had any relation to military uses except, perhaps, the ten million dollars designated for the renovation of ramshackle army barracks in Bolivia. In contrast, of the $2.07 billion in aid provided by the United States to Latin America in 2007, about 45 percent was military aid to Colombia.[5]

The antagonism of the United States toward independent, left-leaning governments in the Western Hemisphere is nothing new. From the 1950s to early 1970s, the branches of the U.S. government that execute foreign affairs—the Departments of State and Defense, plus the CIA—combined forces to destabilize and destroy democratically elected progressive governments in Guatemala, Brazil, the Dominican Republic, and Chile. Then, as now, the United States claimed to be supporting democracy when it was actually ushering in repressive or dictatorial regimes. In 1964, Lincoln Gordon, U.S. ambassador to Brazil in 1964, cabled Washington to brag that he was providing "covert support for pro-democracy street rallies," a destabilizing tactic that directly aided the successful military coup against President João Goulart and the dictatorship that followed. In the 1980s, the United States successfully instigated the Contra war against the Sandinistas while at the same time "promoting democracy" through NED, the National Endowment for Democracy, an organization first used to fund the political opposition in Nicaragua.

Today, more than ever, "democracy building" is the name of the "soft power" or "smart power" game played by the U.S. State Department, the U.S. Department of Defense, and the private corporations that work for them. The Department of Defense, with ten times the budget of the Department of State, has become the major player in defining the rules of democracy because it is spending hundreds of billions of dollars to establish compliant governments in Iraq and Afghanistan. The U.S. military hopes to stimulate obedient forms of pseudodemocratic activity through its "information operations" conducted by the U.S. Central Command in the Middle East. Its funding requests for all the kinds of propaganda necessary to overwhelm the occupied territory—news articles, billboards, radio and television programs, polls, and focus groups—jumped from $110 million in 2009 to $244 million in 2010.[6]

The U.S. government disperses much of the money for "intelligence work," "public diplomacy," "strategic information," and "international development" to private contractors, and many of these have found that "soft power" products are just as profitable as the old "hard power" staples, such as armaments and mercenary soldiers. This phenomenon can be briefly illustrated by the trajectory of DynCorp, which started as an aviation maintenance company serving the U.S. Air Force during the 1950s, and over the next forty years expanded into many other areas of military support, including training paramilitary and police forces in Asia, Africa, and Latin America. In 2010, the company wanted to add to its $3.2 billion annual sales by supplying "information management" and "international development" services, so it acquired the much smaller, but highly experienced Casals and Associates, Inc. This company, headed by a Cuban expatriate, Beatriz Casals, had performed many jobs for USAID and the Department of Defense over the years, including contracts with the anti-Cuban propaganda stations, Radio and TV Martí. One of Casals Associates' brand-new contracts was coordinating CamTranparencia, which is supposed to promote "transparency, anti-corruption and responsibility in Central America and Mexico." In part, the assignment involves supporting political opponents of the revitalized Sandinista government in Nicaragua. A few years earlier Casals had performed a similar function in Bolivia in an effort to undermine Evo Morales's government and help the political opposition. The company distributed $18.8 million in USAID dollars to more than 450 organizations.[7] DynCorp announced that this merger "brings together the complementary skills, experience and capacity of Casals and DynCorp International. . . . They offer a best in class combination of competencies to provide services supporting U.S. defense, diplomacy, and international development initiatives and objectives." There seems to be a very strong future in this kind of economic activity. One week after Casals was purchased by DynCorp, Cerberus Capital, a giant private equity firm, stepped in to buy DynCorp. Cerberus was looking for military security corporations with the most potential for worldwide expansion (at the time of the purchase former U.S. vice president Dan Quayle was in charge of international operations at Cerberus).[8]

Another example of the ways that the military is assuming control over public diplomacy and the strategic manipulation of other cultures can be found at the U.S. Southern Command, based in Miami. At the same time it has been expanding its reach in Latin America with the activation of the Fourth Fleet and the use of seven more air bases in Colombia, SouthCom also named its first director for strategic communication and invented the academic discipline of "Strategic Culture." Anthropologist Adrienne Pine reports that a "nonprofit military-industrial academic complex" has grown up around the U.S. Southern Command headquarters in Miami, where it operates a joint "strategic culture initiative" with Florida International University. Here social scientists and military strategists combine their talents to produce reports on the specific attributes of the cultures of individual Latin American and Caribbean nations. According to Pine, who reviewed their report on Honduras, their investigations did not require much academic rigor: "High-quality research is far less important to the alliance than creating high-quality antidemocratic propaganda to justify the support of the coup-installed government and increased U.S. military presence and aid."[9]

AID that Is Not Aid

While the United States Agency for International Development has distributed assistance to countries around the world for half a century, a large proportion of these programs were directly connected to the hard power of U.S. military counterinsurgency. At its inception, USAID was primarily involved in Vietnam in police training, rural pacification, and overall support for the strategic hamlet system. More recently USAID has developed new methods of putting soft power programs, including democracy promotion, to work in support of military counterinsurgency operations and has taken part in all aspects of pacification in Iraq and Afghanistan. It is also using some of these counterinsurgency techniques in its Office of Transition Initiatives, or OTI, to destabilize governments and provoke regime change in countries where there are no wars being fought. Usually working in conjunction with NED, the OTI works to destabilize and undermine governments that the U.S. government does not approve of. This destabilization is called "democratic transition."

In 2001–02, after Cuba and Venezuela signed the first of their agreements of economic, social, and medical cooperation, the State Department dispatched Otto Reich, who had headed up the first Office of Public Diplomacy in the 1980s, to Venezuela to work with the political opposition and NED operatives on efforts to undermine the democratically elected government of President Chávez. NED had begun preparing the groundwork by abruptly increasing its funding for opposition political activity from $50,000 in 2000 to $340,000 in 2001, and then again to nearly $1 million in early 2002.[10] Lacking originality, the U.S. interlopers and their Venezuelan allies gave the same name to the anti-Chávez coalition that Otto Reich and NED had used for the anti-Sandinista opposition they created in Nicaragua two decades earlier: Coordinadora Democratica. This civilian destabilization was immediately followed by the unsuccessful military/oligarchy coup against Chávez in April of 2002, but the United States was not about to give up. Later in the year, USAID stepped in to assist NED by forming an Office of Transition for

Venezuela. The desired "democratic transition," of course, was the fall of the Bolivarian government that had been winning democratic elections with a high rate of citizen participation and transparency. Over the next eight years, USAID would spend over $50 million on contracts with U.S. private consulting firms, in particular Development Alternatives, Inc., or DAI, which in turn funded and trained over 600 opposition political groups.[11] In 2005, former CIA agent Philip Agee wrote that the United States was following the same pattern of subversion that it had practiced in Nicaragua, Latin America, and the developing world for many decades: "DAI then established an office in Caracas, very possibly as a front for and with personnel from the CIA, while passing as an ordinary subsidiary of a U.S. transnational corporation. In reality, it is a key office of the U.S. embassy disguised as a private company." Even if DAI was not operating as a direct front for CIA personnel, it was certain that the CIA was playing its customary historical "role in supplying secret funds and providing clandestine support"[12] to the forces that wanted to oust Chávez.[13]

DAI has performed contracts for USAID and the Department of Defense all over the world, including extensive work in the "pacification" of Iraq and Afghanistan; in 2008, it took over major USAID contracts for the "democratic transition" process in Cuba because members of Cuban American organizations in Miami, the previous recipients of funding, had been found guilty of widespread fraud and corruption. The following year, DAI operative Allan Gross was arrested in Havana for distributing sophisticated communications equipment to Cuban citizens. Washington-based Cuba analyst Anya Landau French reported that another government contractor told her that "USAID-funded organizations had been sending as many as fifty people a month into Cuba in order to deliver 'technical and financial' assistance to dissident activists on the island."[14]

Cuba, of course, has been the number one target of U.S. harassment ever since its revolution in 1959. But in 2002, at the same time overt U.S. interference was escalating in Venezuela, James Cason was sent to head the U.S. Interests Section in Havana with a new assignment, to directly encourage and support internal destabilization.

Cason recruited a small group of political dissidents and provided them with monetary support and communications equipment, and even traveled throughout the country trying to drum up new recruits. Roger Noriega, assistant secretary of state for western hemispheric affairs in the Bush administration, later revealed that he and his colleagues in Washington had instructed Cason to engage in the most disruptive and outrageous behavior possible. They were hoping he would foment so much "chaos" that the Cuban government would expel him, thus precipitating a complete break in diplomatic relations with the United States.[15] Cuba chose not to kick Cason out of the country, but its reaction against the dissidents who had cooperated with Cason was used by the United States to fuel a rapidly escalating *guerra mediatica*, or "media war," that has never ceased. When Cuba arrested about seventy-five people for taking aid from a foreign power in order to engage in activities harmful to the government (a crime not only in Cuba but also in the United States and most countries of the world), the U.S. State Department and the global corporate media loudly proclaimed that this was a grave assault on democracy, human rights, and freedom of expression.

The Bush administration, with its Western Hemisphere department well stocked with anti-Cuba experts, used the Cuban response to these provocations as the rationale for more funding for destabilization and "regime change." In 2004, the Bush administration created the Commission for Assistance to a Free Cuba to "explore ways the U.S. can help hasten and ease a democratic transition in Cuba," and the following year implemented a number of measures that would make life more difficult for people on the island, including further restrictions on travel, a crackdown on cash transfers by Cuban Americans to their relatives, and making new funding available for disruptive "information warfare" campaigns. To increase international pressure on Cuba, the United States funneled substantial funds to foreign countries; for instance, in 2005 NED paid the governments of Poland, Romania, and the Czech Republic $2.4 million to subsidize anti-Cuba organizations in their nations.[16] In 2006, the destabilization program was augmented with the "Cuba Fund for a

Democratic Future" plan, which allotted another $80 million for anti-Cuba propaganda and for building up opposition forces within the country. To further this effort, in August 2006 the Bush administration tried to sabotage Cuban medical initiatives by launching an unprecedented attack on that nation's humanitarian aid program. The Cuban Medical Professional Parole Program was specifically designed to lure Cuban doctors, nurses, and technicians away from their foreign assignments by giving them special immigration status for entry into the United States. Although the parole law seems to have done little to reduce the effectiveness of Cuba's health missions or increase the rate of defection, it does demonstrate the degree of animosity engendered in the minds of Washington bureaucrats. A U.S. government website claims that this cynical anti-humanitarian measure was permitted because of a Homeland Security statute that "permits parole of an alien into the United States for urgent humanitarian reasons or significant public benefit."

The sabotage aimed at Cuba was directly supported by the actions of the U.S. ambassadors to Venezuela, William Brownfield and Patrick Duddy, who served there between 2004 and 2010. The embassy in Caracas interfered regularly in that nation's internal political matters, cooperated with the Venezuelan opposition groups that were encouraging Cuban medical personnel to desert, and expedited the exit visas for the small number who did leave for Miami. Embassy cables from Venezuela indicated that Barrio Adentro was a primary target of the U.S. disinformation campaigns; these reports ignored the widespread, well-documented improvements in health care and repeated the false and undocumented claims in the opposition press (sometimes funded by the embassy or NED) that "the quality of health care in Venezuela has declined." In 2008, Duddy asked for assistance from U.S. military experts in directing the embassy's "strategic communications" assaults on Venezuelan public opinion. One of his embassy cables, released by WikiLeaks, reads: "Embassy Caracas requests DOD [Department of Defense] support in the execution of its strategic communications plan. The goal for this program is to influence the information environment within Venezuela. . . . DOD support would greatly enhance existing Embassy Public Diplomacy and pro-democracy activities." The vigorous involvement of the ambassadors in destabilization operations was connected to their strong military and national security orientation; earlier in his career Brownfield was political adviser to the commander in chief of the Southern Command during the invasion and occupation of Panama, and both he and Duddy earned degrees in National Security Strategy from the National Defense University. They are representative of a whole cadre of State Department veterans of the Central American wars who have ascended to the most important positions in the U.S. embassies throughout Latin America. Many of them have also served on the Cuba desk in Washington and at the U.S. Interests Section in Havana. Almost all of them share a history of working closely with the Department of Defense, the CIA, the powerful anti-Castro Cuban exile community in Miami, and conservative think tanks such as the Heritage Foundation.[17]

La Guerra Mediatica, *The Media War*

It is well documented that news stories in the U.S. corporate media, as well as many of their associates in other countries, are overwhelmingly negative whenever they report on Venezuela, Cuba, and their ALBA allies.[18] In 2006, just before the the Cuban Medical Professional Parole Program was put into effect, Michael Parmly, head of the U.S. Interests Section in Havana, sent a cable out to the rest of the Latin American embassies, reminding them that they were "always looking for human interest stories and other news that shatters the myth of Cuban medical prowess, which has become a key feature of the regime's foreign policy and its self-congratulatory propaganda."[19] Generally, articles based on diplomatic reports are fed to major media reporters who are accustomed to socializing with embassy and military personnel, and the news tips are published with little or no verification. The media are constantly fed by conservative think tanks, such as the Heritage Foundation, that have close links to the U.S. Defense and State Departments and churn out a steady stream of propaganda about the mounting threats in the Western Hemisphere. They regularly refer to the elected presidents of Venezuela and Bolivia as dictators and push for drastic action with messages such as "State Sponsors of Terrorism: Time to Add Venezuela to the List" and "U.S. Should Reject Illegitimate Election Process in Bolivia."[20]

The progressive governments in the hemisphere feel that they are the victims of a *guerra mediatica* and *terrorismo mediatico* (media war and media terrorism) because the global media offer them absolutely no space to counter these specious accusations. Whereas the corporate news services are telling only the stories that the U.S. government wants told, they have an even more effective way to hurt the images of Cuba, Venezuela, and the ALBA nations: when it comes to Cuban/Venezuelan cooperation and medical internationalism in the region, they do not report the news at all. That is, they can generally be relied upon never to publish or broadcast favorable stories that feature the extraordinary accomplishments in health care and education. The rarity of the positive stories can be illustrated by the U.S. coverage of Haiti's earthquake in 2010. Less than a week after the quake, there was one favorable story, a CNN television report on Cuban doctors by reporter Steve Kastenbaum:

> There are so few places where ordinary Haitians can turn when they are in need of urgent medical care in the center of the city. We came across one: La Paz hospital. It is now being administered by Cuban medical personnel here in Haiti alongside crews from Spain and Latin America. And it is amazing to see. They are giving medical attention—quality medical care—to severely injured people, six to seven hundred patients a day, several dozen surgeries a day. They have three theaters going around the clock, 24-7, and it is one of the only places deep in the city where Haitians can go and be treated and have a reasonable expectation of surviving.

In the months that followed, CNN, even with their high-profile correspondents Anderson Cooper and Sanjay Gupta spending weeks in Haiti and countless hours on television, never once followed up on that report, nor did they visit the Cuban medical installations that were all around them. The major U.S. newspapers were as bad as CNN, or perhaps worse, in their coverage during a two and a half-month period after the quake, according to the research of Emily and John Kirk: "Between them the *New York Times* and the *Washington Post* had 750 posts regarding the earthquake and relief efforts, though not a single one discusses in any detail any Cuban support."[21] The same pattern of neglect continued for many months and confirmed the Kirks' research. When Project Censored named the outstanding stories that were ignored by the major corporate media for the year, one of them was "Cuba Provided the Greatest Medical Aid to Haiti after the Earthquake."

Just about this time, in December of 2010, a few stories about Cuban medical prowess did appear in major media outlets. One Reuters news service story, carried by a number of U.S. newspapers and websites, gave favorable attention to the intensive efforts by Cuban health teams who were leading the fight against the cholera epidemic in Haiti.[22] The tendency spread to Britain with an article by Nina Lakhami in the *Independent*, "Cuba's Doctors Are the Backbone of the Fight Against Cholera in Haiti," that then circulated in a number of newspapers.[23] Shortly thereafter, Ray Suarez of the PBS *NewsHour* devoted two lengthy and mostly favorable reports on Cuba's universal system of health care and the medical education provided at the Latin American School of Medicine.[24] Though these stories may have been aberrations that do not signal any major changes in media coverage, Cuba and Venezuela can still hope that the tide will change. The *guerra mediatica* that is waged against them in order to discredit their societies can only be successful if there are no breaches in the barricades that block the real stories. If accurate information begins to penetrate the mediasphere, the cloud of disinformation released by the U.S. counterinsurgency effort will quickly dissipate and fade away.

12. Practicing Medicine, Practicing Revolution

Above all, try always to be able to feel deeply any injustice committed against any person in any part of the world. It is the most important quality of a revolutionary.

—CHE GUEVARA, letter to his children, 1965

Of all the forms of inequality, injustice in health care is the most shocking and inhumane.

—MARTIN LUTHER KING JR.

The revolutionary doctors and medical students from Cuba and Venezuela and the rest of the Americas—and the nurses, physical therapists, sports trainers, and other skilled technicians who work with them—are offering a serious challenge to the rest of the world. By their daily deeds and commitment to socialist solidarity, they are demonstrating that humanity is capable of delivering medical care to everyone—not in the remote future, but right now—and they are accomplishing this while openly defying the logic of capitalist development that dominates most of the globe. Cuba and Venezuela have demonstrated that a model of comprehensive community medicine, based on over half a century of successful experimentation in Cuba and abroad, can be adapted to the needs of other nations. This is no easy matter, since at the same time they are constructing a universal public system of primary care, advanced care, and preventive medicine they are also training the medical personnel who will sustain that system over the long haul.

The intensive grassroots, democratic participation of the Venezuelan people in the ongoing development of Barrio Adentro has been crucial to the success of the Cuban collaborators; it also has been indispensable in the evolution and deepening of the Bolivarian revolutionary process. For this reason, the Venezuelan experiment is an inspiration to other societies that are trying to invent their own versions of twenty-first-century socialism. Citizens are learning to meet one of their most important social needs by inventing a new logic of health care and education, and in the case of the young campesinos who were my neighbors in Monte Carmelo, they are achieving their goals by doing what in any other circumstances would seem impossible. Graduates of the village's three-room high school and those who completed their secondary studies in the evening classes of the education missions are now students working diligently to complete a rigorous six-year medical program. The crucial element that makes this possible is exactly the one stipulated by Che fifty years ago: "For one to be a revolutionary doctor or to be a revolutionary at all, there must first be a revolution."[1]

Since the doctors and their students are operating within the context of radical social change, it has been possible to develop a unique medical curriculum and communicate scientific knowledge in brand-new ways. The new revolutionary doctors learn the same medical science that is taught throughout the world, only in a formulation that emphasizes the interrelatedness of the various traditional medical sciences and integrates them into broad courses of morphophysiology and morphopathology. In the course of their formal studies, their daily exposure to patients and practical questions of care have habituated them to integrate their growing scientific knowledge with the complexities of diagnosis and treatment. The fact that the students have daily access to extensive DVD material that relates to each formal class, often reviewed in study sessions with other students, gives them multiple opportunities to interpret or reinterpret the meaning of the scientific concepts and their social/medical applications. In the course of their work rotations that begin in the first year, they have intensive experiences with a wide variety of doctors, professors, and tutors that last throughout the entire six-year training period; this exposes them to a depth and range of interpretations of academic material and diagnostic evidence that is not duplicated in the educational experience of privileged first-world medical students.

The new Cuban-Venezuelan system of medical education, Medicina Integral Comunitaria, has taken the concept of apprenticeship and reconfigured it. By working half the day alongside a master/tutor, the apprentice/student learns not only the knowledge and techniques of the specialty, but also the social context and the ways the community can make use of this art. Although the Cuban medical artists are teachers devoted to disseminating the conscientious use of the craft, just as masters have done for centuries, they have a very distinct motivation. Unlike the artisans who formed craft and professional guilds in the past and the wealthy medical associations that control the physician's craft in many parts of the world today, the Cubans have no desire to limit the number of practitioners. Because they are not worried about the possibility of economic competition lowering their earnings and because the ethical standards of their craft require them to treat anyone who is suffering without regard for payment, the members of this revolutionary guild are devoted to multiplying their numbers until they reach all who need their care and support.

All this is possible because the doctors' prestige derives not from high incomes and conspicuous consumption but from the high level of respect they receive from the communities they serve. This respect is generated by the physicians' personal example of selfless service, their willingness to live among the people they treat, their egalitarian approach to their patients, and their interest in promoting consciousness and participation of the community in improving their own health and "wellness." The overwhelming majority of the Cubans who volunteer for this kind of service are not about to be lured away by the monetary rewards promised by capitalist medicine, and this leaves a lasting impression on the people they treat and those who they train. The inspiration the doctors supply has a very practical effect on those who will one day replace them, for they are offering them both the necessary scientific knowledge and the lessons in how physicians ought to behave with patients, interact with communities, and work as a cohesive group. The new guild members must demonstrate considerable individual initiative and personal adaptability in the face of difficult local conditions, but they also have to know how to cooperate. According to the prescription provided by Che in his speech "On Revolutionary Medicine," this blend of creative individualism and social solidarity is absolutely necessary:

> But for this task of organization, as for all the revolutionary tasks, fundamentally it is the individual who is needed. The revolution does not, as some claim, standardize the collective will and the collective initiative. On the contrary, it liberates man's individual talent. What the revolution does is orient that talent. And our task now is to orient the creative abilities of all medical professionals toward the tasks of social medicine.[2]

Medical Practice, Revolutionary Praxis

The manner in which revolutionary doctors and health workers are reproducing themselves and expanding their numbers suggests a path, a model of daily practice and education that leads far beyond the field of health care. The revolutionary doctors, because they are engaged in health care, are *practicing* medicine, but also because they are revolutionaries, are *practicing* the construction of revolutionary society—that is, while they are building they are also acquiring new skills, consciousness, and social behavior. They are engaging in *praxis,* which for Aristotle meant the engagement of philosophical

thought in human activity, and for revolutionary theorists, and especially for Marx, meant the "revolutionary, critical-practical activity"
that is necessary for changing the world. Marx—and for that matter,
Gramsci, Freire, and others who followed him—understood that
humans are not going to transform their societies unless they simultaneously transform themselves by practicing revolutionary behavior,
social commitment, and humanitarian ethics in their everyday lives
and work.

All too often, however, when socialists have taken power and prescribed the parameters of political and economic organizations, they
have produced few working models of the everyday praxis necessary
to create new kinds of human interaction. The "real socialist" world of
the twentieth century—represented in the end by the failed bureaucratic states in the Soviet Union and Eastern Europe—offered few
examples of people engaged in meaningful, productive work in free
and egalitarian settings with their fellow citizens. Nor were there signs
that pointed toward the liberating association of people that the
authors of the *Communist Manifesto* had proclaimed as the goal of revolution: "an association in which the free development of each is the
condition for the free development of all."

One of the key challenges for twenty-first-century socialist revolutions, because they are conscious of the serious shortcomings of twentieth-century revolutions, is to provide daily work and activity that is
functional in an economic and social way but also allows people to
develop more fully as human beings. The notion that Che was
describing, that individuals can liberate and develop themselves more
fully when they are devoted to the full and revolutionary development
of their communities and society, is at the foundation of *medicina
integral*. Throughout most of this book, the word *integral* has been
translated as "comprehensive" because it is the best English word for
indicating that a service or program is wide-ranging and complete.
The word *integral*, however, also signifies complete in the sense of
"whole," as in *pan integral* (whole-grain bread), and thus connotes
how individuals should be treated within the community program.
Doctors, nurses, health workers, and family members are taught to

consider the good health, the holistic health—physical, emotional, social, and spiritual—of each person. Another dimension that concerns the individual is the development of the *medico integral,* the whole and complete doctor, who is expected to exercise, often in the most trying circumstances, a wide range of skills and scientific perception, as well a strong spirit of empathy and solidarity. In this regard, the Cuban physicians and those they train meet the standards of the "five-star doctor": Caregiver, Decision Maker, Communicator, Manager, and Community Leader.[3] These five qualities are deepened by international service and the demands of relating to other cultures, and in the case of those who take on the duties of professor/tutor, their full development is completed with a sixth star: Teacher.

Cuban and Venezuelan medical cooperation, then, is not just about offering better health care, but about preparing people to remake the world. As Hugo Chávez declared in 2004, the time has come not only "to defend humanity" but to "go on the offensive" and "rescue the concept of socialism."[4] Over the next several years, he elaborated on this idea often, explaining that socialism had to be a liberating process that allowed poor and working people to be the protagonists in building a new society and pursuing their own self-development. In one nationally broadcast talk in 2009, he quoted from a letter that the famous Russian anarchist, Peter Kropotkin, wrote to Lenin: "Without the participation of local forces, without organization from below by the workers and peasants themselves, it is impossible to build a new life."[5] For socialist theorist Michael Lebowitz, who has been living in Venezuela and supporting the Bolivarian process for most of the past decade, this marks a return to the broad humanist vision that ought to be the basis of socialist revolution: "The idea of making human development the center of a concept of socialism and stressing that this development occurs only through practice is, in fact, a return to the critical insights of Marx."[6]

New Models of Self-Development
Frighten the North

In the warped view of U.S. government military and political analysts, the new socialist activity in the Americas has taken on the aura of a "super-insurgency."[7] The U.S. animus against all things connected to Cuba and the Castro brothers has existed for fifty years, but over the past decade Washington has extended this paranoid attention to Hugo Chávez. For them, Chávez is a mastermind who has mesmerized the Venezuelan populace and made them hostage to his dictatorial fantasies; furthermore, they believe he is enticing other leaders like Evo Morales and Rafael Correa into practicing the same kind of demagoguery. The counterinsurgency warriors in Washington fail to understand what would be readily obvious if they spent a few weeks or months amid the residents of Venezuela or Bolivia: these people are participants in a popular insurrection against inequality and poverty, and their so-called insurgency is really a grassroots movement of millions of people who are using democratic means to transform themselves and their nation.

There is, of course, another factor looming behind the faulty analysis and projection of evil intentions: Hugo Chávez, Evo Morales, and the Castro brothers are leaders of small countries that are daring to display economic and political independence. The revenues from Venezuelan petroleum are being channeled toward the needs of the people of Venezuela and the Americas rather than toward the banks of the United States, the United Kingdom, Spain, and the rest of the advanced capitalist world. The profits from the newly discovered lithium deposits in Bolivia will, according to Evo Morales, be controlled by the state, not by the biggest multinational corporate investors. Cuba's major asset, the human capital generated by its remarkable education system, is not investing itself in hedge fund and banking activities, but is generously sharing itself with other nations.

The panic at the center of the capitalist world is due to the fact that twenty-first-century socialism is an attractive proposition to many nations. What if South Africa, for instance, which has mineral riches and export revenues comparable to Venezuela's, decided to take control of its economic and social destiny?[8] Most of South Africa's population lives in conditions far more wretched than Venezuela's people did a decade ago, even though it belongs to the same category of "middle income" countries of the world (those with average per capita incomes in the $10,000 to $14,000 range). Though per capita incomes in Venezuela rank near the top of this range (along with the other richest countries in South America: Argentina, Uruguay, and Chile), they are not even close to the high-income status of the advanced industrial countries of Europe, North America, and Asia, which have per capita incomes that are about three times as high. Still, it is evident that this level of affluence, quite modest on a global scale, is sufficient for funding great transformations in social and economic conditions at home and abroad. The first step in the process in Venezuela was difficult politically but simple in its conception: the profits from the extraction of natural resources must be kept at home instead of being sent to corporate and financial centers in the rich nations.

This rearrangement of the rules of the global political economy can produce funds for replicating new models of social production, as is the case with health care linked with Cuban medical cooperation. It is a social invention that is threatening to the global production of social privilege, much as the nationalization of natural resource industries threatens the global appropriation of surplus value. In this case, it undermines the foundations of class-based medicine in developing countries, which until now have mimicked the existing arrangement of medical practice in advanced societies. Professor Julie Feinsilver of Georgetown University has explained why the presence of egalitarian doctors strikes fear in the hearts of entrenched elites in countries that receive Cuban aid:

> Cuban medical diplomacy is a great benefit to the recipient countries, but also a threat. The threat lies in the fact that Cuban doctors serve the poor in areas in which no local doctor would work, make house calls a routine part of their medical practice, and are available free of

charge 24/7. Because they do a diagnosis of the community and treat patients as a whole person living and working in a specific environment rather than just clinically and as a specific problem or a body part, they get to know their patients better. This more familiar approach is changing expectations as well as the nature of doctor-patient relations in the host countries. As a result, Cuban medical diplomacy has forced the reexamination of societal values and the structure and functioning of the health systems and the medical profession within the countries to which they were sent and where they continue to practice. In some cases, such as in Bolivia and Venezuela, this threat has resulted in strikes and other protest actions by the local medical associations as they are threatened by these changes as well as what they perceive to be competition for their jobs. As Cuba's assistance concentrates more on the implementation of some adaptation of their own health service delivery model, the threat will become more widespread.[9]

This threat, which may mildly affect the doctors who are already embedded in health systems that serve the elite, pales beside the greater, more general threat from the Cuban-Venezuelan model. The worldwide extraction of profit by the imperial centers of finance has been practiced for the last five centuries and has always depended on the explicit or implicit use of violence, either by imperialist countries themselves or by comprador classes and the local armies who serve them. Fifty to sixty years ago, it appeared that national liberation movements and guerrilla forces like those that triumphed in Cuba were the primary impediment to the global expansion of capitalism, and the imperialist countries developed their doctrines of counterinsurgency in response. Now that the "insurgents" are creating *el ejercito de batas blancas,* the army in white jackets, Washington strategists are totally unprepared and unequipped mentally to mount a defense. The Cuban medical missions, the graduates of ELAM, the Henry Reeve Brigade, and other students in training do not represent a military threat at all, for they think of themselves as "an army of peace," as Dr. Yonel told me in Caracas in 2004. At the same time they represent a moral and ethical weapon that is striking at the hollow core of capitalist values.

First of all, the insurgents subscribe to a philosophy of political economy that calls for diverting profits that support overconsumption in the north toward the satisfaction of basic human needs in the south. Secondly, they question the sincerity, or at least the efficacy, of the kind of humanitarianism that is currently in vogue in the north. The non-government organizations, or NGOs, that are spawned by the hundreds of thousands in the rich regions of the world are proving to be a weak solution, and sometimes a detriment, to solving the social problems and health care needs of the poor nations of the earth. Unni Karunakara, himself a member of Médecins Sans Frontières (an NGO that does accomplish useful work in Haiti and elsewhere), delivered a scathing rebuke to other NGOs that operated in Haiti for an entire year after the earthquake of 2010. He demanded to know why they could not even organize themselves to deliver clean water to the Haitian people. "Why have at least 2,500 people died of cholera," he wrote, "when there are about 12,000 NGOs in the country?"[10]

Worldwide, the NGOs say they want to help the poor, but few of them send qualified health personnel like the Cuban brigades who are equipped, scientifically and psychologically, to dedicate themselves to living and working among the poor and learning from them about the most urgent health needs of their communities. According to Daniel Esser, expert on international aid at Columbia University, most foreign donors do not take this kind of approach: "When funds are committed, neither multilateral agencies nor foundations seem to take into account what recipients in Africa, Latin America, and the poorer parts of Asia consider the most severe causes of ill health."[11] Another scholar, William Easterly of New York University, author of *The White Man's Burden,* criticizes first-world aid programs in general for forcing their agendas on the poor, but has singled out organizations like the World Bank in particular. Typical of the bank's approach was insisting on more funds for HIV/AIDS in Malawi even though other donors were already meeting this need, and then cutting funds for nutrition and general reform of the nation's health care delivery system.[12] Although first-world countries have showered charitable and development dollars on AIDS to the neglect of public health programs, their gains in fighting the progress of HIV infection are sometimes fleeting. Uganda had bragged in the past about making great progress with its AIDS prevention programs, but recent United Nations statistics show that for every 100 people put on treatment in Uganda, 250 others are newly infected.[13]

Over the past three decades, the ascendancy of neoliberalism and the extreme emphasis on market solutions for every human need have seriously warped international approaches to health care. As vast sums of surplus wealth accrued to the richest investors in the advanced capitalist countries, philanthropic institutions and private NGOs greatly increased their involvement in global health care issues and other humanitarian endeavors.[14] The super-rich, who meet at the World Economic Forum in Davos, Switzerland, to send up cheers for "creative capitalism" and "social entrepreneurship," annually choose a group of "Young Global Leaders." In 2010, these sixty people decided they were numerous enough to announce their own "People's Plan of Action" that would "fight the key challenges of poverty around the world." Typical of the so-called young global leaders listed on the World Economic Forum website was Nicky Newton King, deputy chief executive officer of the Johannesburg Stock Exchange.[15]

This kind of intense involvement of the richest private economic interests has shifted the focus of medical aid away from "horizontal" integrated public health programs that emphasize primary care and prevention (programs traditionally backed by the World Health Organization and the Pan American Health Organization), and toward top-down, vertical campaigns that concentrate on quick-hitting, publicity-generating campaigns against individual diseases. Although some of these programs have been effective at times, they often detract from primary health delivery, in particular by hiring away the few health care providers who are available to work in the public health system. Ill-conceived intervention has aggravated the biggest deficit faced by the poorest developing countries in regard to health care: the scarcity of doctors, nurses, and health workers of all kinds.

The wealthiest countries have, on average, about twenty-eight doctors per 10,000 people, while the least developed countries, such as Ethiopia, Kenya, Rwanda, Sierra Leone and Somalia, have fewer than one for every 10,000 people. While lack of financial resources and educational facilities is a key factor, the power of the brain drain that empties from south to north is equally detrimental. More than half of the health workers originally born in Kenya currently work abroad according to a British health care advocacy group. Ghana, though substantially better off economically than Kenya, wasted $52.5 million from 1998 to 2002 training health professionals who ended up working in the United Kingdom. This was a bargain for the United Kingdom since it would have had to spend much more to train the same number of people at home.[16]

On the other end of the spectrum, in the country that spends far more per capita on health care than any other nation, the future of primary care and truly universal medical attention is surprisingly bleak. In 2008 only 2 percent of all medical students in the United States planned careers in primary care internal medicine, down from 9 percent in 1990.[17] Consequently, students graduating from U.S. medical schools were filling only 42 percent of the postgraduate residencies offered in family medicine; foreign graduates took most of the rest of the places, a factor that also contributes to the global brain drain. Much of the decline in interest in primary care is due to one of the destructive market mechanisms that exercise so much influence over the U.S. medical system. According to the Association of American Medical Colleges, the average educational debt in 2009 for graduates who took out loans to attend school (the great majority) was huge, $156,456. No wonder, then, that students were flocking to careers in orthopedic surgery, dermatology, and plastic surgery that offered average annual earnings of $400,000, and rejecting family medicine and internal medicine because those careers paid less than half as much.

Cuba and Venezuela, which together have a population of 39 million, currently have more students in medical school, about 73,000, than the United States, with a population of over 300 million.[18] All the doctors in Cuba and Venezuela are educated for free, some even receive stipends for living expenses, and almost all of them will do a three-year specialty in family medicine after graduation, after which they may pursue a second specialty. The United States has generally had 68,000 to 70,000 students enrolled in all of its medical schools at any one time, and about 16,000 graduate each year. If 2 percent are specializing in family medicine, this would only amount to 320 of them.

There are, of course, many potential students in the United States who would like to enter the field of medicine for ethical and humanitarian reasons and work in their home communities, especially if they were offered an annual salary approaching $200,000. If the medical schools decided to increase their enrollments in order to produce more family doctors, it would be rather easy to put them to work. This would require a few guarantees that advanced capitalist countries can certainly afford: free medical school education, universal and egalitarian insurance coverage for their patients, and adequate medical facilities in the poorer parts of cities and rural areas. The fact that this very wealthy country is willing to deny the opportunities that could effectively deliver health care to its own people, while also sabotaging the efforts of poorer nations to build new kinds of public primary care medical systems, is one of the great scandals of twenty-first-century capitalism.

Seremos Como El Che: *We Will Be Like Che*

Fortunately, as a consequence of the determination, experience, and collaboration of Cuba and Venezuela, twenty-first-century socialism continues to fight on behalf of comprehensive community medicine. Many countries that are already receiving aid from Venezuela or instruction from Cuban internationalists would like to form their own corps of dedicated community physicians. One unique quality of the Cuban-Venezuelan collaboration, and the smaller experiments in medical education that Cuba is launching in other countries, is that the medical students are not separated from their homes and neighborhoods, thus making it much more likely that graduates will fit into the long-term health plans of their communities and their nation. The former health minister of East Timor, Rui Araujo, hopes that the ethos of medical service demonstrated by the Cubans in his country will help combat the brain drain and encourage new doctors trained by the Cubans to keep working at the village level.[19] This will be difficult to achieve, however, unless this impoverished and war-torn nation finds financial support for a universal primary health care system and decent conditions of employment for its health care workers. It is possible that some funding for new health care systems and doctors' salaries could come from an outside source, such as Australia, which has discussed entering into joint ventures with the Cubans to help East Timor.

In Haiti, Brazil has already made a series of firm commitments to work with Cuba in designing and constructing a new national health care program that will eventually be administered and staffed by the Haitians themselves. Cuba's minister of health, Dr. Jose Ramon Balaguer, spoke at a ceremony celebrating one of these agreements in Croix du Bouquets, Haiti, in March of 2010, and gave lofty praise to the potential inherent in this kind of cooperation: "What would the world look like if all men and women lent their skills and solidarity like those of the Henry Reeve Brigade? It would be a world full of peace, of love—a different world."[20] On the other side of the globe, a Christian health aid worker expressed similar feelings about the Cuban Medical Brigades in East Timor: "It is the friendship of the poor and not the rich, the weak and not the strong. It is strange that the best example of Christian behaviour and good deeds comes from a secular country. This is an intriguing mystery; one that deserves pondering by those of us who profess to be Christian."[21] This is really not so mysterious if one knows two things. One, Che once wrote:

At the risk of seeming ridiculous, let me say that the true revolutionary is guided by great feelings of love. . . . In these circumstances one must have a large dose of humanity, a large dose of a sense of justice and truth in order to avoid dogmatic extremes, cold scholasticism, or an isolation from the masses. We must strive every day so that this love of living humanity is transformed into actual deeds, into acts that serve as examples, as a moving force.[22]

And two, for decades Cuban schoolchildren have been beginning each day by saying: *Seremos como el Che*: We will be like Che. Today these schoolchildren have grown up and devoted themselves to intrepid missions in some of the most destitute parts of the world, and medical students in Venezuela and the internationalist volunteers from the Latin American School of Medicine are following them. They are walking in the footsteps of the *guerrillero heroico*, the heroic guerrilla leader, by becoming *médicos heroicos* and donning their white jackets in a new kind of army, *el ejército de batas blancas*. October 8, the day that Che Guevara was assassinated in Bolivia, is celebrated as El Día del Guerrillero Heroico in Cuba. Since 2009, the same day has also been celebrated in Venezuela, but there it is called El Día del Médico Integral Comunitaria. In this case, the new "comprehensive community doctors" are being celebrated as the heirs to Che's legacy, and Che himself is being acknowledged as the prototypical heroic physician.

In Cuba and Venezuela, Che serves as the ideal of the conscientious internationalist who fights for humanity and, by dedicating himself to revolutionary activity, changes himself in the process but never loses his individuality or distinct identity. Behind this ideal, and busy building reality, are the thousands of committed physicians and medical personnel—brave, resourceful, empathetic, imaginative, and persevering individuals themselves—who for the past fifty years have been the ones who actually charted the course of revolutionary health care, developed the concepts and innovations in training, adapted to severe economic constraints when necessary, and proceeded to construct new systems of health care.

The accomplishments of the revolutionary doctors and their internationalist coworkers have an importance that goes far beyond the provision of health care and the alleviation of suffering. The combination of medical service and medical education in Venezuela serves as an example of what the fusion of the Cuban and Bolivarian Revolutions can achieve, and demonstrates that the most difficult and challenging kinds of work can be organized on the basis of universal and egalitarian guidelines. Socialists of the twenty-first century, and some of us who were socialists in the twentieth century, have known for some time that revolutionary praxis requires "telling by doing." It is rather easy for intellectuals and political leaders to tell campesinos and urban workers that they ought to create productive cooperative workplaces. It is much more difficult for any of us to summon the energy, master the necessary skills and interpersonal relations, and then find the revolutionary situation that will permit us to build these new social and economic structures.

Today the lessons learned in the area of medicine can be applied to other kinds of work and social service. This may mean adopting relevant portions of the master–apprentice model or breaking down the barriers between theory and practice. Unnecessary walls that divide manual and intellectual labor—for instance, between technical experts and production workers in agriculture, construction, and manufacturing—will fall when the manual laborer works in a congenial, egalitarian environment where "the free development of each is the condition for the free development of all."[23]

The cooperative efforts of Venezuela and Cuba, highlighted by their medical programs, are serving as the models for humanitarian relationships and fair economic exchange between the nations of the south. Revolutionary doctors and health workers, through their example and their commitment to constructing a new kind of socialism in a new century, are providing convincing proof that another world, a better world, is possible.

Notes

1. WHERE DO REVOLUTIONARY DOCTORS COME FROM?

1. "Hoy somos un ejército de batas blancas que dará salud y un poco más de dignidad a nuestros pueblos." Dr. Katia Millaray, quoted in Rodolfo Romero Reyes, "Le nacen retornos a la salud publica cubana y latinomeri-cana," http://www.almamater.cu, 2007.
2. Emily J. Kirk and John M. Kirk, "Cuban Medical Aid to Haiti," Counterpunch.com, April 1, 2010.

2. SOLIDARITY AND INTERNATIONALISM

1. "Haitian Fact Sheet," issued by *MEDICC Review*, http://www.medicc.org, January 15, 2010. The website follows up with ongoing information on Haiti.
2. Leticia Martinez Hernandez, "Haiti: U.S. Doctors Working in Cuban Hospitals," *Granma*, February 5, 2010.
3. Leticia Martinez Hernandez, "Vaccination Campaign in Haiti," *Granma*, February 17, 2010.
4. Leticia Martínez Hernández, "Cuban Doctors in Haiti: "The worst tragedy is not being able to do more,'" *Granma*, January 18, 2010.
5. Tom Jawthrop, "Cuba's Aid Ignored by Media?," Al Jazeera, February 19, 2010.

6.   Paul Farmer, "Further Interview Excerpts from ¡Salud!," www.salud.org, February 2006.
7.   Ernesto de la Torre Montejo, Salud para todos, si es posible. La Habana: Sociedad Cubana de Salud Publica Seccion de Medicina Social, 2004, 260.
8.   Emily J. Kirk and John M. Kirk, "Cuban Medical Aid to Haiti," Counterpunch.com, April 1, 2010.
9.   Gail A. Reed, "Where There Were No Doctors: First MDs Graduate from Latin American Medical School," MEDICC Review, August–September 2005, http://www.medicc.org,
10. "Haiti's Health Crisis Grows Worse with Political Turmoil," Paul Jeffrey, ACT International, Dateline ACT (Action by Churches Together), May 26, 2004, http://act-intl.org/news/dt_nr_2004/dthaiti0204.html.
11. Radio Guantánamo, "Destacan humanismo de la enfermería cubana en Haití," February 28, 2010.
12. "Cuban health professionals are 'absolutely' important for Haiti: WHO official," United Nations Radio, February 17, 2010.
13. Conner Gorry, "Interview with Dr. Patrick Dely: Part I," and "Part II," Field Notes from MEDICC, www.mediccglobal.wordpress.com, April 5 and April 20, 2010.
14. W. T. Whitney Jr., "First There Is God and Then the Cuban Doctors," People's World, May 3, 2010.http://peoplesworld.org.
15. W. T. Whitney Jr., "Cuba, ALBA Send Aid Directly to Haiti," People's World, May 3, 2010.http://peoplesworld.org.

3. CREATING TWO, THREE . . . ONE HUNDRED THOUSAND CHE GUEVARAS

1.   Ernesto Guevara, "Create two, three . . . many Vietnams, that is the watchword," The Tricontinental, magazine of Organization of Solidarity with the Peoples of Asia, Africa, and Latin America, April 1967.
2.   Enrique Milanés León, "Fidel, Chief Inspiration for Cuban Medical Cooperation," Granma International, November 5, 2008.
3.   Jean Friedman-Rudovsky and Brian Ross, "Peace Corps, Fulbright Scholar Asked to 'Spy' on Cubans, Venezuelans: U.S. Embassy Official's 'Spy' Request Violated Long-Standing U.S. Policy," ABC News, February 8, 2008.
4.   Kevin Hall, "In Bolivia, Push for Che Tourism Follows Locals' Reverence," Knight-Ridder, August 17, 2004.
5.   Nick Buxton, "Searching for Che," Red Pepper, October 25, 2007.
6.   Hedelberto Lopez Blanch, Historias Secretas De Medicos Cubanos, Ediciones La Memoria, Centro Cultural Pablo de la Torriente Brau, 2005.

7.   Argiris Malapanis and Roman Kane, "Mandela: "Cuba Shared the Trenches with Us,'" *The Militant*, 59/39, October 23, 1995.

8.   Margaret Blunden, "South-South Development Cooperation," *International Journal of Cuban Studies* (June 2008).

9.   Luis Jesús Gonzalez, "Concluye VII Encuentro Hemisférico de Lucha contra los TLC," *Trabajadores*, April 11, 2008; Gail Reed, "Cuban Doctors around the Globe, More Doctors for the World," *MEDICC Review*, April 14, 2008.

10. Hedelberto López Blanch, "La escuela cubana de Medicina en Zanzíbar," *Juventud Rebelde*, June 23, 2009.

11. "Cuban Doctors Serving Poor to Be Expelled from Honduras," NotiCen: Central American & Caribbean Affairs, http://www.allbusiness.com, September 1, 2005.

12. Diane Appelbaum and Hope Bastian Honduras, "Cuban-Trained Garifuna Doctor Story of American Honduran Cuban Cooperation in Honduras," *Cuba Health Reports, MEDICC Review*, September 2008.

13. "Guatemala Plans to Send More Medical Students to Cuba," *Granma*, January 31, 2008.

4. MEDICINE IN REVOLUTIONARY CUBA

1.   "Salud en Tiempo. 1970-2009," Ministerio de Salud Publica, Cuba, 2010, http://files.sld.cu/dne/files/2010/11/salud-en-el-tiempo-2010.pdf. Figures for United States and Europe derived from OECD ratios of practicing doctors per 1000 citizens. Nearly 25 percent of Cuba's physicians were working abroad.

2.   Ileana del Rosario Morales Suárez, MD, MS, José A. Fernández Sacasas, MD, MS, and Francisco Durán García, MD, "Cuban Medical Education: Aiming for the Six-Star Doctor," *MEDICC Review*, 10/4 (Fall 2008).

3.   Ibid.

4.   Ibid.

5.   Ernesto de la Torre Montejo, *Salud para todos, si es posible*. La Habana: Sociedad Cubana de Salud Publica Seccion de Medicina Social, 2004, 50.

6.   World Health Organization and the United Nations Children's Fund, "Report of the International Conference on Primary Health Care, Alma-Ata, USSR, 6–12 September 1978," WHO Health for All series, no. 1, Geneva, 1978.

7.   "Primary Health Care Comes Full Circle. An Interview with Dr. Halfdan Mahler," *Bulletin of the World Health Organization*, October 2008.

8.   Howard Waitzkin, MD, PhD, Karen Wald, Romina Kee, MD, Ross Danielson, PhD, Lisa Robinson, RN, ARNP, "Primary Care in Cuba: Low- and High-Technology Developments Pertinent to Family Medicine,"

Division of Community Medicine, University of New Mexico, Family Practice Center, 1997.

9.   Morales Suárez et al., "Cuban Medical Education."

10.   Louis A. Perez Jr., *Cuba: Between Reform & Revolution*, New York: Oxford University Press, 1988.

11.   "UNDP Publishes Report on Human Development and Equity in Cuba," *MEDICC Review,*3/2(2000).

12.   Clarivel Presno Labrador, MD, MPH, and Felix Sansó Soberat, MD, "20 Years of Family Medicine in Cuba," *MEDICC Review*, 6/2 (2004).

13.   André-Jacques Neusy, MD, and Bjorg Palsdottir, MPA, "A Roundtable of Innovative Leaders in Medical Education," *MEDICC Review*, 10/4(Fall 2008).

14.   Gail Reed, "Cuba's Primary Health Care Revolution: 30 years on," *Bulletin of the World Health Organization* 86 (May 2008).

15.   Indira A. R. Lakshmanan, "As Cuba Loans Doctors Abroad, Some Patients Object at Home," *Boston Globe,* August 25, 2005.

16.   Patricia Grogg, "CUBA: World Class Pharma that Puts People First," *International Press Service,* December 1, 2009.

17.   Figures for the year 2008, from World Health Organization, http://www.who.int (accessed 2010).

18.   Gail Reed, "Generating Appropriate Technologies for Health Equity," *MEDICC Review* 11/1 (Winter 2009).

5. BARRIO ADENTRO

1.   Quoted in Argiris Malapanis and Camilo Catalán, "Cuban Doctors in Venezuela Operate Free Neighborhood Clinics," *The Militant,* October 23, 2003.

2.   Eugenio Radames Borroto Cruz, MD, Ramon Syr Salas Perea, MD, "National Training Program for Comprehensive Community Physicians, Venezuela," *MEDICC Review* 10/4 (Fall 2008).

3.   Ibid.

4.   Claudia Jardim, "Prevention and Solidarity: Remedies for Democratizing Health in Venezuela," Voltaire.net, October 13, 2004.

5.   Moses Naim, "The Venezuelan Story: Revisiting the Conventional Wisdom," Carnegie Endowment for International Peace, April 2001.

6.   Mike Whitney, "Interview with Eva Golinger," Counterpunch.org, December 18–20, 2009.

7.   Mark Weisbrot, Rebecca Ray, and Luis Sandoval, "The Chávez Administration at 10 Years: The Economy and Social Indicators," Center for Economic and Policy Research, February 2009.

8.   Bernardo Alvarez, "Revolutionary Road," *Foreign Affairs*, July–August 2008.

9.   Weisbrot, "The Chávez Administration at 10 Years."

10. Mark Weisbrot and Luis Sandoval, "Update: The Venezuelan Economy in the Chávez Years," Center for Economic and Policy Research, February 2008.

11. Peter Maybarduk, "A People's Health System in Venezuela," *Multinational Monitor,* December 1, 2004.

12. Argiris Malapanis and Camilo Catalán, "Cuban Doctors in Venezuela Operate Free Neighborhood Clinics," *The Militant,* October 23, 2003.

13. Ibid.

14. Associated Press, "Cuba and Venezuela Deepen Ties with Medical-Oil Swap," Wednesday, July 13, 2005.

15. Figures from CIA country studies for 1998. For 2008 the studies showed that Venezuela's per capita GDP was $12,000, much greater than the low-income countries, but still a far cry from a truly rich country like the United States, where per capita income was $46,000.

16. In everyday practice, when Venezuelans refer to the small neighborhood consulting offices of Barrio Adentro I as *consultorios* or *ambulatorios,* they could mean any of the walk-in primary care facilities no matter whether they are newly constructed or renovated spaces. However, *consultorios populares* is the name used by the Barrio Adentro Mission for the consulting offices that are newly created by the program, and *ambulatorios* has been retained for the consulting offices that were built many years earlier by former governments. When they say that a consulting office is a "modulo," however, they only mean the newly constructed red brick octagonal structures.

17. Municipalities in Venezuela differ greatly. Some can be large urban areas with 1.5 million people, such as the Libertador Municipality of Caracas, which is more or less the equivalent of a city borough like Brooklyn, New York. Other municipalities are the equivalent of rural counties in the United States, where 50,000 or fewer people can be spread out over a large geographical area, as is the case with Andres Eloy Blanco, the municipality where I lived in the state of Lara.

18. The development of Barrio Adentro was pretty much complete at this time, since in 2011 the government cited virtually the same number of *consultorios populares* (6,712) that were operational.

19. President Hugo Chávez speaking on national television about the accomplishments of the Bolivarian Revolution on February 2, 2011.

20. "Dictan auto de detención a constructores que abandonaron obras en hospitales," *Correo de Orinoco,* February 10, 2011.

21. Kiraz Janicke, "Venezuelan Health Spending among Highest in the Americas," Venezuelanalysis.com, February 20, 2008.

22. Tamara Pearson, "82% of Venezuelans Use Public Health System," Venezuelanalysis.com, June 8, 2009.

23. "Salud de Ninez," Sistema Integrada de Indicadores Sociales de Venezuela, Ministerio de Poder Popular de Planificacion y Financias, Gobierno de Venezuela, http://www.sisov.mpd.gob.ve/indicadores.
24. Charles Briggs and Clara Mantini-Briggs, "Confronting Health Disparities: Latin American Social Medicine in Venezuela," *American Journal of Public Health* 99/3 (March 2009).

6. WITNESSING BARRIO ADENTRO IN ACTION

1. Peter Maybarduk, "A People's Health System in Venezuela," *Multinational Monitor,* December 1, 2004.
2. It was only after reading Enrique Ubieta Gómez's *Venezuela Rebelde* a year later (2009) that I realized Ariel was Ariel Hernandez, twice Olympic and twice world amateur champion, whom Ubieta had interviewed extensively for his book in 2005.
3. Enrique Ubieta Gómez, *Venezuela Rebelde,* 114-15.
4. Robin Nieto, "Inside the Barrio: Venezuelan Health Care Takes Off," Venezuelanalysis.com, August 5, 2004.
5. Ubieta Gómez, *Venezuela Rebelde,* 215-18.
6. These government doctors did not work for Barrio Adentro but in the public service established by previous governments that are often working at cross purposes with Bolivarian programs. These doctors and the Venezuelan doctors in private practice in Sanare refused to collaborate with the Cuban doctors.

7. NEW DOCTORS FOR VENEZUELA

1. Peter Maybarduk, "Cultural Change and Community Care," *Multinational Monitor*, December 1, 2004.
2. Enrique Ubieta Gómez, *Venezuela Rebelde,* 201-4.
3. Argiris Malapanis and Camilo Catalán, "Cuban Doctors in Venezuela Operate Free Neighborhood Clinics," *The Militant*, October 23, 2003.
4. Author's interview with Ruth Martinez, coordinator of Mission Sucre Health Education for the state of Miranda, at the Universidad Bolivariana de Venezuela, Caracas, spring 2009.
5. Eugenio Radames Borroto Cruz, MD, and Ramon Syr Salas Perea, MD, "National Training Program for Comprehensive Community Physicians, Venezuela," *MEDICC Review* 10/4 (Fall 2008).
6. André-Jacques Neusy, MD, and Bjorg Palsdottir, MPA, "A Roundtable of Innovative Leaders in Medical Education," *MEDICC Review* 10/4 (Fall 2008).

7. Ubieta Gómez, *Venezuela Rebelde*, 206.
8. Ibid., 205.
9. My compilation of a detailed chart by Dr. Pedro Diaz of the Barrio Adentro National Academic Coordinating Committee, which appeared in Borroto Cruz, "National Training Program for Comprehensive Community Physicians, Venezuela."
10. Ibid., 40.
11. Ibid., 41.
12. Ibid., 40.
13. Ubieta Gómez, *Venezuela Rebelde*, 211.
14. Dr. Charles Boelen, *The Five-Star Doctor: An Asset to Health Care Reform?* Monograph on the Internet (Geneva: World Health Organiza-tion, 1993), available at http://www.who.int.
15. Ubieta Gómez, 202.
16. Aday del Sol Reyes, "Creo en los caballeros andantes de la solidaridad," an interview with Enrique Ubieta Gómez, my translation, *Cubasí*, February 7, 2007; available at http://www.rebelión.

9. REVOLUTIONARY MEDICINE IN CONFLICT WITH THE PAST

1. "Fuga de Medicos," *Tal Cual* (Caracas), March 27, 2009.
2. Author's interview with Arelys and other MIC medical students, Monte Carmelo, February 8, 2008.
3. Paco Ignacio Taibo II, *Ernesto Guevara: Also Known as Che* (New York: St. Martin's, 1997), 307.
4. When I attended the Encuentro de Artistas y Intelectuales en Defensa de Humanidad in Caracas in December 2004, President Hugo Chávez attended the proceedings on four different days and talked openly about his socialist views. One afternoon and evening, he spent seven hours answering the questions of a wide variety of leftists from Latin America and the rest of the world concerning his views, the global political situation, and historical and philosophical influences on his thinking. He proved himself remarkably patient and well-read, and although he has a reputation for dramatic rhetoric in his public speeches, his behavior was very professor-like (of course, he had been a professor at the national military college before he got involved in politics). He listened to countless inquiries, often prefaced by long-winded proclamations from members of the audience of more than 300, and took careful notes on each question and the identity of the questioner. After each five questions, he would formulate his answers in concise fashion, seldom straying off the subject. He insisted on staying until every participant had an opportunity to ask a question or make a short statement.

5. Enrique Ubieta Gómez, *Venezuela Rebelde: Solidaridad vs. Dinero* (La Habana: Editorial Abril, 2006).

6. These statistics were cited by participants during a meeting of local school teachers and political activists with sociologist Carlos Ganz at the MonCar women's cooperative in the state of Lara, March 2008.

7. "Situación Actual de los Médicos venezolanos de barrio adentro," Aporrea.org, January 12, 2009.

8. Grace Livingston, "Venezuela tries to put Chávez to the test: Opposition raises petition for mid-term referendum on the president's revolution," *The Guardian*, August 16, 2003.

9. Argiris Malapanis, *The Militant*, May 5, 2004.

10. "Noticiario," *El Diario de los Deltanos*, September 2, 2005, 2.

11. Ubieta Gómez, *Venezuela Rebelde*, 225.

12. Jeroem Kuiper, "Barrio Adentro II: Victim of Its Own Success," Venezuelanalysis.com, July 28, 2005.

13. Radio Nacional de Venezuela, December 9, 2008.

14. "Denuncian atropellos: Asociación de Médicos por Venezuela alerta para impedir acciones contra Barrio Adentro," Aporrea.org, February 25, 2009.

15. The pro-Chávez website of news and opinion, *Aporrea,* had been full of health care discussions and revelations of problems as they arose in Barrio Adentro. While the Cuban medical workers have been reluctant to criticize their hosts, a report by the Cuban Venezuelan friendship committee, delivered by Cuban vice minister of health Aldo Muñoz in 2008, mentioned that bureaucratic inattention and unwarranted delays by private contractors were preventing Barrio Adentro from meeting all its projected goals on time.

16. Julie M. Feinsilver, "Cuban Medical Diplomacy," in Mauricio A. Font, ed., *Changing Cuba, Changing World* (New York: CUNY Bildner Center for Western Hemisphere Studies, 2008), 283.

17. Maria C. Werlau, "Cuba's Cash-for-Doctors Program: Thousands of Its Health-Care Missionaries Flee Mistreatment," *Wall Street Journal,* August 16, 2010.

18. "Sources with Miami's massive Cuban exile community say that around 2,000 physicians and other health care personnel have defected since 2006 and requested visas to come to the United States. Of that number, 500 came through Venezuela and just in the last year, about 200 arrived in Miami." *Merco Press,* January 9, 2010.

19. Ibid.

20. *Salud!,* directed by Connie Field, http://www.saludthefilm.net/ns/cuba-and-global-health.html. 2006.

21. ABN, Bolivarian News Service, "Leiany Galano: Médicos cubanos se entregan a la causa latinoamericana," October 8, 2009.

22. Katherine Edyvane, "Timor, Cuba, and the Making of a Medical Superpower," *The New Internationalist*, October 2008.

10. THE BATTLE OF IDEAS AND THE BATTLE FOR OUR AMERICA

1. *Report of the Select Committee on Assassinations of the U.S. House of Representatives* (Washington, DC: United States Government Printing Office, 1979).
2. Cintio Vitier, "Resistance and Freedom," 1992, trans. in *Boundary 2* 29/3 (Durham, NC: Duke University Press, Fall 2002).
3. Interview with Abel Prieto by Alejandro Massia and Julio Otero for *Tiempo de Cuba*, November 7, 2004.
4. Mauricio A. Font, "Cuba and Castro: Beyond the Battle of Ideas," in Mauricio A. Font, ed., *Changing Cuba, Changing World* (New York: CUNY Bildner Center for Western Hemisphere Studies, 2009).
5. Ibid.
6. U.S. State Dept., "A Review of U.S. Policy toward Venezuela: November 2001-April 2002," Report Number 02-OIG-003, July 2002, http://oig.state.gov/documents/organization/13682.pdf.
7. I was in Caracas when Chávez mentioned moving toward socialism for the first time. The three quotations come from Marta Harnecker, "Latin America and Twenty-First Century Socialism: Inventing to Make Mistakes," *Monthly Review*, July–August 2010. She cites Tomas Moulian, *Twenty-First Century Socialism: The Fifth Way*, 2000.
8. These figures come from the CIA's *2010 Country Guide*, which can be found online.
9. Douglas Lefton, "Nicaragua: Health Care under the Sandinistas," *Canadian Medical Association Journal* (March 15, 1984).
10. Eugenio Taboada and Richard M. Garfield, "Health Services Reforms in Revolutionary Nicaragua," *American Journal of Public Health* 74 (1984), 1138–44.
11. Hedelberto Lopez Blanch, "Gobierno Sandinista revertir el deterioro económico y social," rebelión.org, July 26, 2010.
12. Mike Gonzalez, "Latin America's Forgotten Marxist," *International Socialism*, July 2, 2007.
13. Jose Mariategui, "Aniversario y balance," *Amauta*, no. 26 (September 17, 1928).
14. John Riddell cites interview with Marcelo Saavedra Vargas in "From Marx to Morales: Indigenous Socialism and the Latin Americanization of Marxism," mrzine.monthlyreview.org, June 17, 2008.
15. Santa Cruz right-wing groups were dominated by white Europeans with ties to neo-Nazis; youth organizations mounted frequent racist attacks

against indigenous people, and sometimes displayed swastikas and fascist slogans.

16. Cubainformacion TV, "Brutal agresión contra médicos cubanos en Bolivia," August 14, 2008.

17. Dr. Ernesto de la Torre Montejo et al., *Salud para todos: Sí es posible* (La Habana: Sociedad Cubana de Salud Publica, 2005), 260.

18. Paul Farmer, "Who Removed Aristide?" *London Review of Books,* April 15, 2004. In a response to the article, Canadian researcher Anthony Fenton reported that Sam Goff, Brian Concannon, and Father Luis Barrios took part in an International Action Committee investigation into the Dominican Republic's role in the coup. They were able to determine that the Haitian rebels—former military and FRAPH members—were incorporated into the Dominican army in 2000. These paramilitaries were initially trained by the Dominicans, and funded by the International Republican Institute and the National Endowment for Democracy.

19. Enrique Ubieta Gómez, *Venezuela Rebelde: Solidaridad vs. Dinero* (La Habana: Editorial Abril, 2006), 306.

20. "Australia and Cuba Look to Aid Cooperation," http://www.cubaheadlines.com, June 10, 2010.

11. THE WAR ON IDEAS:
THE U.S. COUNTERINSURGENCY CAMPAIGN

1. The phrase "War of Ideas" may have originated with a Heritage Foundation article in 1993 that declared the U.S. government must keep committing itself to the "War of Ideas" even though the Cold War had been won. James Glassman was an innovator in "negative branding," especially at *Tech Central Station*, a corporate service and website that specialized in "journo-lobbying." This is writing propaganda stories for corporations and then passing them off as legitimate journalism. Tech Central Station was well known for working with energy giants such as Exxon-Mobil to disseminate pseudo-scientific reports that disparaged valid scientific articles on global warming and environmental destruction.

2. Spencer Ackerman, "Future of Public Diplomacy Unsettled at State," *Washington Independent,* February 17, 2009.

3. The U.S. State Department was making similar statements around this time. "Venezuela's neighbors are bothered by close ties between the Venezuelan and Cuban governments and their potential dangers to democracy," State Department spokesman Adam Ereli said in May 2004.

4. Colonel Max G. Manwaring, "Venezuela's Hugo Chávez, Bolivarian Socialism, and Asymmetric Warfare," October 2005, Strategic Studies Institute, U.S. Army War College. Many of his ideas were shared by mili-

tary and neoconservative participants at the conference "Charting New Approaches to Defense and Security Challenges in the Western Hemisphere," co-sponsored by the Latin American and Caribbean Center of Florida International University and the Strategic Studies Institute of the U.S. Army War College in Coral Gables, Florida, March 9–11, 2005.

5. "Venezuela provides 4 times the assistance of the US in Latin America," according to Quixote Center, http://www.quixote.com, August, 29, 2007, citing figures that appeared in the *Miami Herald*.

6. Walter Pincus, "Pentagon Reviewing Strategic Information Options," *Washington Post*, December 27, 2009.

7. Nestor Garcia Iturbe, "Hitting Cuba through Bolivia, USAID Objective: Bolivia," *Global Research*, http://www.globalresearch.ca, May 29, 2008.

8. Juan O. Tamayo, "Colombia: Private Firms Take On U.S. Military Role in Drug War," *Miami Herald*, May 22, 2001.

9. Adrienne Pine, "Coup University: SOUTHCOM and FIU Team Up on Counterinsurgency," http://upsidedownworld.org, November 10, 2010.

10. Eva Golinger, "Washington Increases Clandestine Ops Against Venezuela," *Postcards from the Revolution*, http://chávezcode.com, November 11, 2010.

11. Eva Golinger, "Agent Captured in Cuba," *Postcards from the Revolution*, http://chávezcode.com, December 13, 2009.

12. Philip Agee, "Use of a Private U.S. Corporate Structure to Disguise a Government Program," venezuelanalysis.com, September 8, 2005.

13. There is no way to know how much the U.S. has been spending over and above the publicly acknowledged NED and USAID funds on destabilization operations against Venezuela, Cuba, and their allies. The historical record in Latin America (for instance, Chile, 1970–73) would indicate that U.S. intelligence agencies are definitely funding various kinds of covert operations and economic sabotage. The secret funds available are considerable, even if they amount to just a small fraction of the immense expenditures devoted to U.S. intelligence worldwide. By 2010, the amount spent for all global spy operations had grown so large that the *Washington Post*— the U.S. newspaper with perhaps the closest relationship to Pentagon, CIA, and military circles—said it "was beyond control," with a minimum budget of $75 billion, 'but the total size is considerably larger according to intelligence experts interviewed." Dana Priest and William M. Arkin, "A Hidden World, Growing Beyond Control," *Washington Post*, July 19–20, 2010. Of this, two-thirds, or more than $50 billion, was part of the "black budget" of the Department of Defense Intelligence Agency according to experts at *Aviation Week*, leaving about $25 billion for the CIA.

14. Anya Landau French, "Hillary Clinton Got It Wrong: We're Sabotaging Ourselves with USAID Program in Cuba," *Havana Notes*, April 13, 2010, www.havananote.com.

15. Noriega was interviewed on a WQBA radio show in Miami, *What Others Do Not Say*, May 20, 2010.

16. Hernando Calvo Ospona, "The CIA's Successors and Collaborators," *Znet*, August 10, 2007, quoting Laura Wides-Munoz, Associated Press, December 29, 2006.

17. Examples of Washington's destabilization/anti-Cuba/national security specialists heading up the diplomatic corps in Latin America: Hugo Llorens, a Cuban exile, became ambassador to Honduras in 2008; he previously had worked with Otto Reich in the Bush administration and was director of Andean affairs at the National Security Council in 2002 during the coup attempt against Venezuelan president Hugo Chávez. His predecessor, Charles Ford, was transferred to the U.S. Southern Command in Florida to assist in "strategic advising" to the Pentagon on Latin America. Robert Callahan became ambassador to Nicaragua in 2008. He had worked as a military–State Department liaison and an aide to Ambassador John Negroponte when the latter was coordinating support from Honduras for the Contra war against the Sandinistas. Paul Trivelli, his predecessor, specialized in antagonizing the government of Daniel Ortega and went on to serve as civilian deputy and foreign policy adviser to the U.S. military's Southern Command in Miami. Other Central America appointments in 2008: Robert Blau, formerly sub-director of Cuban affairs at the Department of State in Washington and political director at the US Interests Section in Havana, became second in command at the U.S. embassy in El Salvador; Stephen McFarland, ambassador to Guatemala, had previously been second in command at the U.S. embassy in Venezuela and director of Cuban affairs at the State Department. James Foley, who served as ambassador to Haiti from 2003 to 2005 and oversaw the removal of President Aristide by U.S. troops, previously worked at NATO headquarters in Brussels. After Foley left Haiti, he became the deputy commandant and international affairs adviser at the National War College in Washington. In Bolivia, interference from the U.S. embassy diminished after 2008, when President Evo Morales kicked Ambassador Philip Goldberg out of the country for conspiring with secessionist forces; Goldberg had helped mastermind the secession of Kosovo from Serbia in the 1990s. The man left in charge, John S. Creamer, chargé d'affaires, had earned a master's degree in national security strategy from the National Defense University. In Washington, P. J. Crowley is the principal spokesperson for the State Department, the assistant secretary for the Bureau of Public Affairs. He previously served in the Air Force for twenty-six years, retiring as a colonel in 1999, and his area of expertise was national security.

18. For example, FAIR, Fairness and Accuracy in Reporting, showed that there is much more negative coverage of Venezuela than Colombia in regard to

human rights by four major U.S. newspapers. "Human Rights Coverage of Venezuela and Colombia Serving Washington's Needs," February 2009; Justin Delacour, "Framing Venezuela: The U.S. Media's Anti-Chávez Bias," *Counterpunch,* June 1, 2005.

19. WikiLeaks, Michael Parmly cable from Havana U.S. Interests Section, June 6, 2006.

20. Ray Walser, "State Sponsors of Terrorism: Time to Add Venezuela to the List," Heritage Foundation, January, 20, 2010; James M. Roberts and Gonzalo Schwarz, "U.S. Should Reject Illegitimate Election Process in Bolivia," Heritage Foundation, December 4, 2009.

21. Emily J. Kirk and John M. Kirk, "One of the World's Best Kept Secrets," *Counterpunch,* April 1, 2010. Stories unreported in 2010: "Cuba Provided the Greatest Medical Aid to Haiti after the Earthquake," *Project Censored,* http://www.projectcensored.org, December 2010.

22. Pascal Fletcher, "Cuban Medics a Big Force on Haiti Cholera Front Line," Reuters, December 3, 2010.

23. Nina Lakhami, "Cuba's Doctors Are the backbone of the Fight against Cholera in Haiti," *The Independent,* December 27, 2010.

24. Ray Suarez, "Debt-Free Doctors Part of Cuba's Foreign Policy Strategy," PBS *NewsHour,* December, 22, 2010.

12. PRACTICING MEDICINE, PRACTICING REVOLUTION

1. Che Guevara, "On Revolutionary Medicine," address to the Cuban Militia, August 19, 1960.

2. Ibid.

3. As described by Dr. Charles Bohlen of the World Health Organization. See chapter 7.

4. At the Encuentro de Defensa de Humanidad, Caracas, December 2004, attended by the author.

5. Quoted in Marta Harnecker, "Latin America and Twenty-First-Century Socialism: Inventing to Avoid Mistakes," *Monthly Review* (July/August 2010). This essay is one of the best introductions to understanding the various currents, new and old, that contribute to contemporary socialism.

6. Michael Lebowitz was interviewed by Srećko Horvat during the Subversive Film Festival and conference on socialism, Zagreb, Croatia, May 1-25, 2010.

7. The description "super-insurgency" originated with a U.S. military theorist (see previous chapter), but it is not commonly used in U.S. foreign policy statements or by other right-wing scholars. For me, however, it nicely sums up the approach of the United States and other imperialist forces, which cannot help but treat any challenge to their

hegemony, no matter how peaceful and beneficent, as a rebel insurgency against imperial rule.

8. This is, after all, very much the kind of path that would have appealed to Nelson Mandela, one very distinct from the current direction of the South African political economy that seems to be creating ever more misery for the majority as well as a few new African billionaires. Twenty-first-century socialism in South Africa might have even more momentous effects on the whole of Africa than it is having in Latin America.

9. Julie M. Feinsilver, "Cuba's Medical Diplomacy," in Mauricio A. Font, ed., *Changing Cuba, Changing World* (New York: CUNY Bildner Center for Western Hemisphere Studies, 2008), 284.

10. Unni Karunakara, "Haiti: Where Aid Failed," *The Guardian,* December 28, 2010.

11. Daniel E. Esser, "More Money, Less Cure: Why Global Health Assistance Needs Restructuring," *Ethics & International Affairs* 23/3 (Fall 2009).

12. William Easterly, "World Bank AIDS Drive Crowds Out Other Health Programs—but Fails to Make Progress on AIDS," http;//www.aidwatchers.com, May 1, 2009. Although Easterly puts too much emphasis on free market economic activity as a solution, his criticisms of the ineffectiveness of paternalistic aid programs are often on the mark.

13. Donald G. McNeil Jr., "At Front Lines, AIDS War Is Falling Apart," *New York Times,* May 9, 2010.

14. NGOs are the seventh largest engine of economic activity in the world, generating $1.3 trillion annually and employing over 45 million people, according to the head of the Rockefeller Brothers Fund, who got his information from Johns Hopkins University studies. I suspect this figure includes all activities funded by religious charities and performed by their members, so certainly most of it cannot be attributed to the generosity of the super-rich. Stephen Heintz, "The Role of NGOs in Modern Societies and an Increasingly Interdependent World," Annual Conference of the Institute for Civil Society, Zhongshan University, Guangzhou, China, January 14, 2006.

15. From "Young Global Leaders," World Economic Forum, www.wefor.org.

16. "Health Workers and the MDGs," Health Poverty Action, undated, http://www.healthunlimited.org

17. Carla K. Johnson, "U.S. Medical Students Shunning Primary Care," *Associated Press,* September 9, 2008.

18. In round figures, 30,000 in Venezuela, 29,000 Cubans and 24,000 foreign students in Cuba. This does not include several thousand medical students studying traditional medicine at the elite universities in Venezuela. The U.S. estimate, also in round figures, approximates the average number of medical students in attendance each year over the past decade. The United States would probably graduate a few thousand more students each year

since its students are in a four-year program rather than a six-year program.

19. Tim Anderson, "Solidarity Aid: The Cuba-Timor Leste Health Programme," *International Journal of Cuban Studies*, December 2008.

20. Conner Gorry, "Trilateral Accord Signed to Rebuild Haitian Public Health System," *MEDICC Review*, mediccglobal.wordpress.com, March 30, 2010.

21. Anderson, "Solidarity Aid."

22. Che Guevara, "From Algiers, for *Marcha*," *Marcha*, March 12, 1965, repr. as "Socialism and Man in Cuba"; this version is from the *Che Guevara Reader* (New York: Ocean Press, 2005).

23. This challenge is particularly dear to me because my "hometown" in Venezuela, Monte Carmelo, is still a farming village. Many young people are going to evening classes in Mission Sucre—computers, nursing, teaching, law—but will not necessarily find employment in these areas. Very few are studying agroecology, a new course that has been added, even though they are surrounded by their own farming families and plots of land. Monte Carmelo is a place that has a wonderful cooperative tradition that goes back more than thirty years, with a strong base of campesino experience in cooperative organization, sophisticated farming techniques, and a deep understanding of egalitarian self-organization. What does not exist here (or elsewhere in the country) is a rational training program linked to a national program to consolidate land—there needs to be a way to start seventeen- and eighteen-year-olds working half a day in the fields, half a day in the classroom or laboratory setting, alongside master farmers who will not only teach them agricultural skills but also the proper patterns of daily work that make physical perseverance both productive and enjoyable. This should not last for a few months, but for a matter of years (say three or four) and be subsidized as necessary. The object on the economic side will be production of more and healthier food, and on the human side the production of a new kind of agroecological campesino farmer, *el campesino integral comunitario*, who in the long run will be accorded as much dignity and community respect as his medical counterpart.

Index